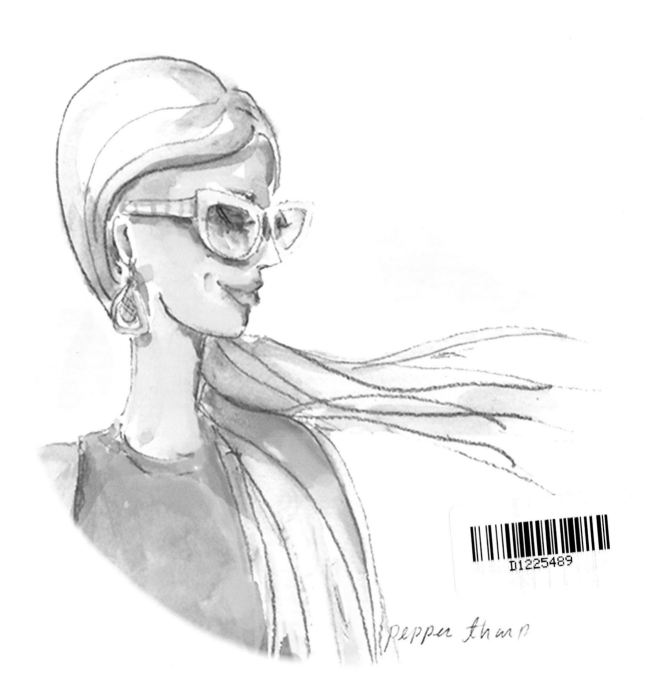

pepper thump

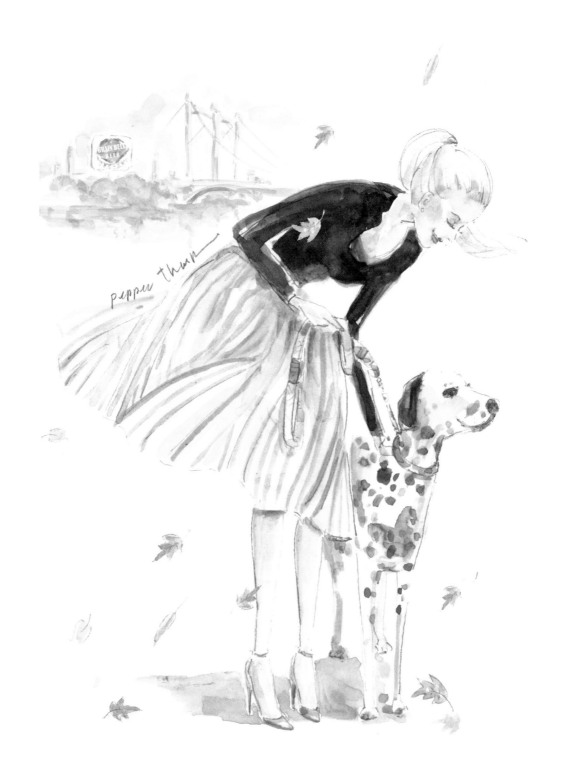

pepper thump

GOING GRAY
BEAUTY GUIDE
50 GRAY8 GOING GRAY STORIES

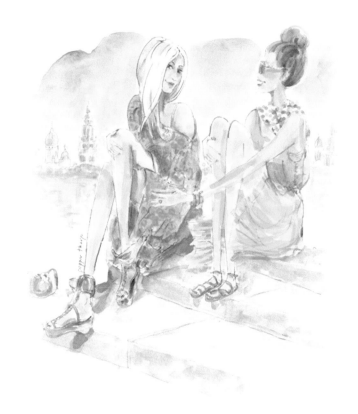

JAN WESTFALL ROGERS

dear graylicious readers

a gray8 big thank you to all the graylicious women
who shared their pictures, stories, and wisdom.
Women will be forever inspired—because of you!

ISBN 978-0-9907219-6-3 (paperback)
ISBN 978-0-9907219-1-8 (e-book)

going gray beauty guide
http://www.goinggraybeautyguide.com/
GGG Going Gray Beauty Guide https://www.facebook.com/GGG.GoGrayGuide
GGG Going Gray Guide https://www.facebook.com/groups/1578474939074185

Jacket design by: Cathy Helms Avalon Graphics LLC
Book design by: eBook DesignWorks

GOING GRAY
BEAUTY GUIDE

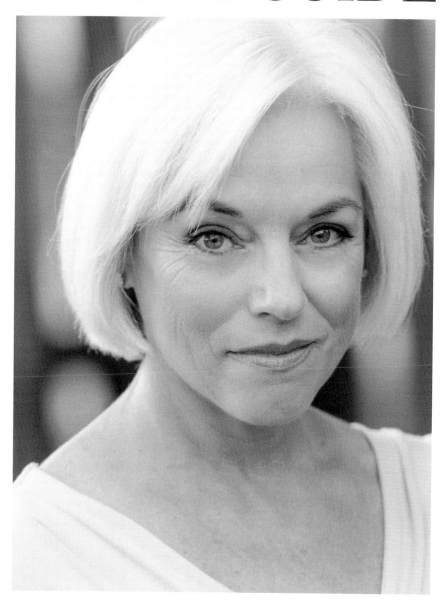

dedication

I dedicate this book in loving memory of my sister Sharon Annette Westfall, who did not get to discover her graylicious self. But, because of her, I discovered mine. I would also like to dedicate this book to my sisters, Barbara, Susan and Lisa, my best friend Shirley, my two daughters, Mistydae and Cheyenne, and granddaughters Bryn and Madison. And last but not least, to my graylicious husband Dale, who has been nothing short of a gift for the past 40 years.

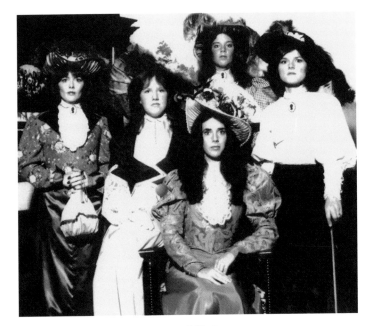

The Westfall Sisters
L-R: Sherry, Lisa, Susie (sitting), Barbara, and Jan (far right).

a gray8 inspiration

My gray8 Aunt Ruby was born in 1912, and is 103 years old. Her mother used to say she was "as tough as a pine knot." Ruby pays her own bills, showers on her own, and cleans her own place. She still wears makeup and gets her hair permed and styled. As far as going gray Ruby says, "Don't try and suit other people, you can't do that, always do what makes 'you' feel good."

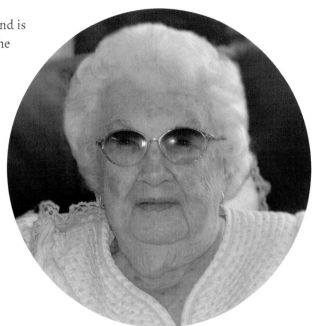

Contents

gray8 beginnings **11**

  graylicious ride 12

  introduction 13

  do you lose your identity when you go gray? 18

  a man's point of view. 19

  your unique color combination 20

  gray8 color combo's 22

ditching the dye **24**

  the long & short of it 25

  what's the best way 2 go gray? 26

  skunk stripe 30

  buzz cut - transition 31

  cold turkey pixie cut – transition 32

  cold turkey length – transition 33

  feathering – transition 34

  highlights/lowlights – transition 35

  gray8 before & after pictures 38

gray8 gray hair **40**

  10 gray8 reasons 2 go gray 41

  10 steps 2 gray8 silver hair 42

  10 gray8 products 4 shine 44

  10 gray8 products 4 style 45

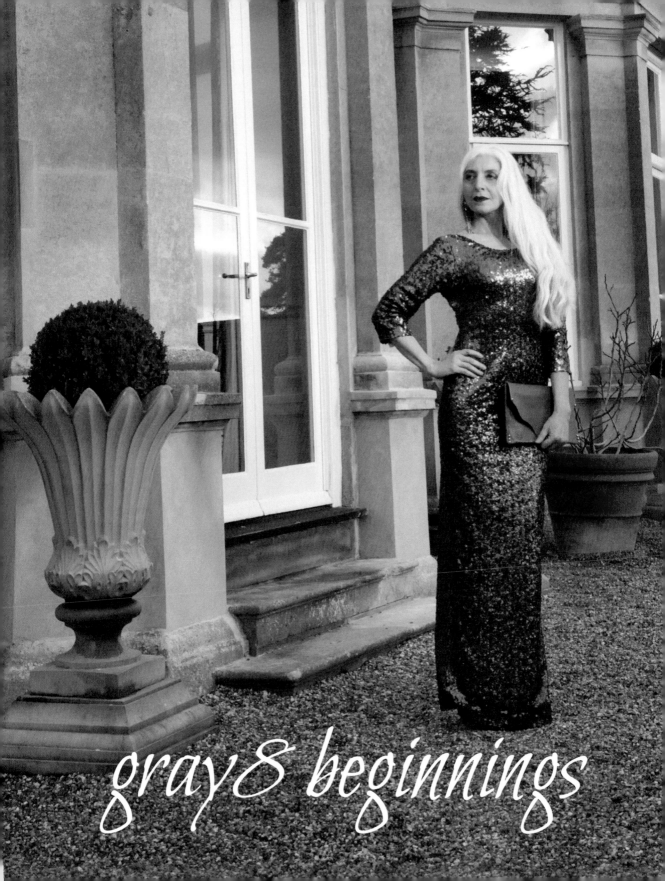

gray8 beginnings

graylicious ride

I was thinking about going gray, but what would people say?
    Should I seek approval or live my life my way?
Tired of coloring; the money and time...
    Planning hair appointments; around occasions of mine.
Going through a transition is no easy fate...
    Some comments will be negative, some comments will be great!
It starts with a skunk stripe that magically appears...
    Perhaps a hair-crayon will make it disappear!
How do I transition with dignity and grace?
    Highlights, cold turkey, a buzz cut with no trace?
Long hair or pixie, whatever I decide...
    I'll do what's best for me on this graylicious ride.

Poem by: Jan Westfall Rogers

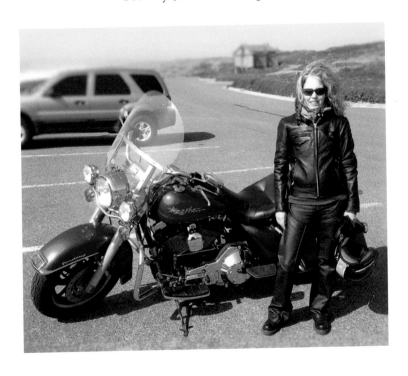

introduction

GOING GRAY BEAUTY GUIDE
50 GRAY8 GOING GRAY STORIES

GGG Going Gray Beauty Guide is specifically designed for women who want to GO GRAY, are GOING GRAY, or, have already GONE GRAY! Here you will find gray8 tips and techniques on hair, skin, makeup, wardrobe, and more. Having gray hair is gray8, and is the NOW color in hair! Having gray hair has nothing to do with age or looking old, and we are determined to change your "old way of thinking!" In the past, gray hair was often associated with the image of a "little old gray haired lady." But today vibrant women everywhere are changing the way we look at gray hair. So hold on to your seats, because the new age of gray is happening now!

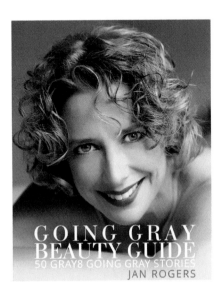

STEPPING OUTSIDE OF THE (DYE) BOX

Stepping outside the box, or going against the norm, is not always the easiest thing to do. But today, millions of women are doing just that! So, why do we dye our hair? For fun? To appear more youthful? Media pressure? Or purely out of a habit that was formed hundreds of years ago? Whatever the reason, leave it up to the baby-boomers to try and squash it! We don't know all your going gray stories, but wanted to share a handful with you, in the hopes that you too, will discover your true graylicious self!

YOUR HAIR - YOUR HEAD - YOUR LIFE!

When you decide to go gray, you will be surprised at how important YOUR HAIR suddenly becomes to everyone. I'm sure you've heard the expression, "Everyone's got an opinion." Well, you will soon find out that it's true! LOL! Nancy Naysayers seem to appear out of nowhere! But, before you grab that bottle of hair color remember this; youth does not come in a bottle of dye, if it did... we would all get in line! The fact of the matter is; not everyone in life is going to like the exact same things as you do - hair color included! Going gray is simply a choice. Give yourself permission to go gray. Beauty goes far beyond the color of a person's hair. Choosing your own route (root) in life can be very empowering!

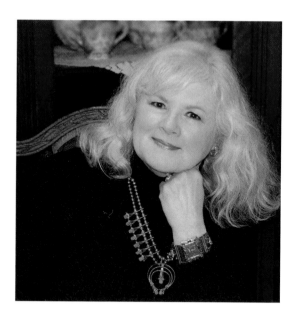

ABOUT ME

I have spent most of my life working in fashion and cosmetics, starting out from behind the cosmetic counter in 1978, and eventually climbing the corporate ladder for three divisions of May Department Stores as: Estee Lauder Beauty Advisor and Counter Manager/Department Manager for Cosmetics, Handbags, and Accessories/Cosmetics Area Sales Manager/Cosmetics Assistant Buyer/and Senior Assistant Buyer for Women's Shoes. I have bought cosmetics and shoes for sixteen department store locations, helped open new doors (stores), organized hundreds of cosmetic events, created cosmetic visual presentations, worked with vendors, set cosmetic standards, and have been honored to hire, train, and manage hundreds of absolutely amazing Cosmetic Beauty Advisors/Consultants throughout the years. I attribute my achievements and awards in cosmetics to strong management skills, being a good listener, and surrounding myself with great talent. Even when I left cosmetics to open my own Bed & Breakfast, I somehow managed to keep "one foot in the door," doing Estee Lauder freelance makeup artistry and promotional work, along with fragrance and jewelry modeling.

Since cosmetics has always been a big part of my life, it seemed only fitting that I decided to go back to school in 2010 at age 57 to get my Managing Esthetician License. I am sure they will always remember the "lady with the gray hair." I passed three Ohio state tests with flying colors, two written (Esthetics/Salon Management), and one practical. My Esthetics credentials include:

- Licensed Managing Esthetician State of Ohio/Tennessee

- Licensed Skincare/Licensed Makeup Artist

- Advanced Facial Treatments/Body Spa Treatments/Relaxation Massage/Hair Removal

- Physiology/Histology/Anatomy/Chemistry/Bacteriology

- Ohio State Board Sanitation/Sterilization/OSHA Safety

GGG GOING GRAY BEAUTY GUIDE

http://www.goinggraybeautyguide.com

GGG Going Gray Beauty Guide https://www.facebook.com/GGG.GoGrayGuide

GGG Going Gray Guide https://www.facebook.com/groups/1578474939074185

Jan Westfall Rogers: Author, Licensed Makeup Artist, (ESTM) Licensed Managing Esthetician, Makeup Junkie, and Baby Boomer. PEACE!

MY GOING GRAY STORY

My going gray story has nothing to do with allergies, being authentic, spending money, bad dye jobs, or time spent in the chair. In fact, I just stumbled upon it - quite by accident!

Although my going gray process was painless, the year 2003 was full of pain. I was on a going gray journey, and didn't even know it! It was as if, I had just woken up one day with white hair. I had spent the year taking care of my oldest sister Sherry, who was 51, and dying of Lupus. Everything about that year broke my heart. We were only seventeen months apart in age and grew up as best friends. I think when we go through something so terrible, we are given a set of blind folders (to help protect us); so we can do what needs to be done. After she passed that January in 2004, at the age of 52, I looked in the mirror at myself and started shaking my head, wondering where all this white hair had come from. But I was full of grief and accepted my new look and dove into my work, doing anything and everything I could to keep my mind busy. One day, I picked up Sherry's old recipe box and started going through it. I gathered up all her best recipes, and asked everyone I knew for theirs, and used them to write my Bed & Breakfast Cookbook, "Don't Forget the INNgredients!" in my sisters memory. I will always be grateful for all the time we had together as sisters and best friends; I will never stop missing her.

Going gray, for me, wasn't something I had planned, or even thought about, so, although I embraced it at the time, I did not acknowledge the process internally. I continued to wear my hair white for a few years, and then decided to have a few lowlights put in. Not because I didn't like my white hair (because I did), I was just looking for a change and thought maybe that was the change I needed. I loved my new lowlights, but six months later, not so much! My white hair was slowly disappearing and I wanted it back. So I started my going gray journey once again, but this time I do remember; it was a conscious decision now, unlike the first time. Fortunately for me, I still had a lot of my white hair mixed in with the lowlights, (she had used my white hair as the highlights), so it didn't take long before the color faded and I was on my way to graylicious hair once again!

I grew up in a musical family and was the second of the five "Westfall sisters." My dad started playing his three dollar guitar, when he was only twelve, and my mother started singing on the radio at age sixteen. Dad taught mom to play bass guitar, and, for 62 years, they made beautiful music together. Of course, it didn't stop there; mom taught each of her five daughters to harmonize! I sang lead, so, I have lots of memories of starting out in the wrong key and everyone laughing, except mom!

My husband and I graduated from the same high school in Wadsworth, Ohio. Many years later, our two daughters graduated from there as well! I have three grandkiddos and two Shih-Tzu's. In 1990, my husband and I started restoration on a dilapidated 1890 Historic Victorian home and turned it into an "Award Winning" Bed & Breakfast. We received several awards throughout the seventeen years of its operation, and were recognized by the city, for the "Significant Contributions to its Beautification, Restoration, and Preservation."

After writing a cookbook for our B&B, I always assumed a future book might entail writing about Bed & Breakfasts! Never once did it enter my mind that I would be sitting here writing a book about GRAY HAIR, but I am so glad I did! All in all, I have been blessed with gray8 friends and family, and have enjoyed a full and rewarding graylicious life.

GRAY8 TIPS & TECHNIQUES

I have tried to keep my hair regime as simple as possible, but have come to the conclusion that I love hair products way too much! Since I received my Esthetician/Aesthetician License, I am privy to professional haircare products, and now there is no stopping me! I'm like a kid in a candy store and love trying out new products.

I wash my hair twice a week with DevaCurl No-Poo and follow-up with DevaCurl One Condition. I like changing products out every now and again, but always stick with a sulfate-free shampoo. I always wash my hair in cool water, as I believe it helps maintain my natural oils, and adds shine. After I wash my hair, I lay a microfiber towel or tee-shirt on my shoulders. While my hair is soaking wet, I apply a small amount of Redken Extreme Anti-Snap (to repair and strengthen my hair). Then I add a small amount of DevaCurl Supercream for extra moisture, shine and frizz control. Then I scrunch it, and leave it be.

Some of my other favorite go-to products for frizz and shine are Redkin Outshine 01, and Pureology Colour Stylist Cuticle Polisher. For second and third day hair, I occasionally use DevaCurl Styling Cream. I find that adding water to a very small amount of product does the trick. I am not into using anything that makes my hair feel crunchy, funky, sticky, or stiff.

When I was attending Esthetics school, I used a blow-dryer and flatiron daily. After several months, the heat turned my hair light blonde! (And no, blondes do not have more fun!) I used a professional-grade flatiron, but it didn't have a temperature control. Now I don't use a blow-dryer or flatiron, and let my hair air-dry naturally. Recently I dug out my mom's old sponge rollers which help smooth and lift the hair. I use a wide-toothed comb and Widu Brush on my hair. In the shower I use a Wet Brush.

To brighten my white hair, I use Pureology Purifying Shampoo with zero sulfates, once every two weeks. It is a clear shampoo as I don't use a purple shampoo. I just mix a small amount with my regular sulfate-free shampoo to avoid drying. Following this hair regime keeps my hair nice, white, and bright.

At night, I lay a large satin scarf (that my mother gave me) across the top of my pillow to prevent frizz and breakage.

After going graylicious, I have made only a few minor changes to my wardrobe colors. The colors I didn't like with my brown hair, I still don't like, i.e. (gold/rust/yellow/yellow-orange/yellow-green). I wear certain cream tones easily, avoiding yellow undertones. Since I have brown eyes and brown in my hair, I continue to wear black/brown chocolate/brown easily, but stay away from red-browns and yellow-browns. I am a creature of habit, and know what I like and don't like when it comes to color, and prefer the richness of deep bold colors. My new favorite color is red-orange!

Makeup is another one of my big downfalls! I am a makeup junkie! How could I not be after being in cosmetics for so many years and becoming a Licensed Makeup Artist? I am always updating my cosmetics, which pretty much keeps me from needing a complete overhaul! LOL! Makeup colors are determined by skin color, hair color, and eye color, along with the skins undertones, so, as an Esthetician, I have made the necessary changes along the way.

When it comes to jewelry, I prefer silver, white gold, and platinum over yellow gold, (just like I always have). I do however wear a few sentimental yellow-gold pieces. My wedding band is both colors, so I have the best of both worlds! I also enjoy wearing vintage Native American Jewelry.

A TIDBIT ABOUT ME

Going to Esthetics school at age 57 was indeed a challenge. I had to learn words like Sternocleidomastoideus. What? All I want to do is give a facial! First I had to learn how to pronounce the 21 letter word, then spell it, know its location on the body, what it was, and, what it did, (muscle of the neck that lowers and rotates the head), now on to the next word. I got this!

do you lose your identity when you go gray?

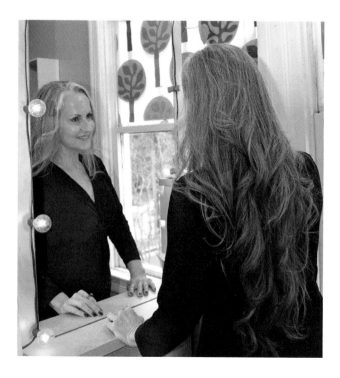

Year after year, we see the same person in the mirror, or so it seems. For the most part, we see ourselves from the waist up, or from whatever angle the bathroom mirror allows, and, if something's a little off, we tend to blame it on our hair. We begin to think, maybe we need a change in hair color, or perhaps highlights will do the trick, so off to the salon we go. There they carefully apply a bottle of youth—I mean hair dye, and POOF, just like magic, we look younger. Or do we? Some seem to think so. But the truth of the matter is—we don't.

Do you lose your identity when you go gray? Yes and No. You certainly alter it, just like you do when you go from straight to curly hair, long to short, or go from dyed dark hair to being a blonde. Often we hear the saying, "It's just hair," but, for most of us, hair seems to matter, and has a lot to do with how we perceive ourselves. If you have always identified yourself with long brown hair, looking in the mirror with short gray hair or short blonde hair will definitely be a jolt to your system; you will be doing a lot of double takes for a while! It will take time and patience to adjust to the new you, it's not going to happen overnight, but eventually it will become the new norm. As we travel through life our identities are constantly changing. The lists of changes we make are endless! The best thing to do is sit back and enjoy your graylicious ride through life!

a man's point of view

BY DALE ROGERS

Going gray was something I never thought too much about. I would wake up with a few gray hairs here and there, and, eventually, the brown disappeared, and the silver took over. It never occurred to me to color my hair, although I know some men do.

Going gray for a man is very much accepted in today's society. I was not told that I would look old; no one stared at me, I was not frowned upon, nor did I receive any negative comments. I also did not ask for anyone's approval, worry about how I looked, or concern myself with what others might think about my gray hair.

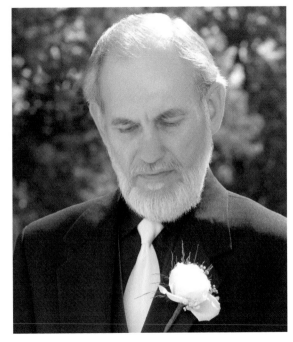

Hopefully someday, going gray for women will also become the norm. Meanwhile, it is important for husbands, family, and friends to get on board and be supportive. The color of a woman's hair has little to do with who she is as a person. If you need to question her gray, then it becomes more about you and less about her. I feel very fortunate to be growing old together with my graylicious wife!

your unique color combination

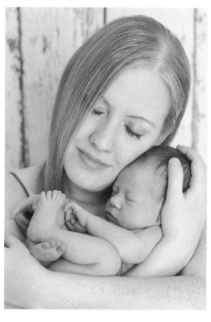

GGG wants every woman to know she is graylicious, no matter what shade of gray, mix of gray, or amount of gray she may have in her hair. It's about setting yourself free from the dye. It's about re-discovering your inner beauty. It's about celebrating who you are, and being comfortable in your own skin. It's about redefining society's perception of beauty. It's about setting real examples for generations to come. It's about choice!

Transitioning, or showing your unique colors, is not always about having all gray hair. You may not have any gray, or you may have very little gray, which brings me to the question, "Unless you are coloring for fun, why are you coloring your hair?" On the flip side of that, you may have a ton of gray hair, and just aren't ready to show the world yet. I get that, too! My 88 year old aunt Thelma NEVER showed the world! She came into this world with dark brown hair, and left it with dark brown hair! LOL! But if YOU are ready to take a leap of faith, I highly doubt that you will be disappointed in what Mother Nature has in store for you!

Gray hair comes in an assortment of shades, not just the "lighter shade of gray," that many associate with gray hair. For years, I thought the darker color at the back of my hair was my natural dark brown. Then, upon closer inspection, I realized it also included charcoal gray! My daughter Cheyenne is 38 and has been dye-free for three years. When you look at her picture holding her daughter, you may or may not, catch a glimpse of the silver sparkles running throughout her hair. She is sporting red hair with her own natural highlights, and it's not costing her a penny! Genetics play a major role in "when" and "how" we gray! Everyone will gray differently; that's what makes having gray hair so unique! By going natural, you will have a front row seat to watch all your color combinations unfold. Someone may have the same color as you, but NO ONE—will have the exact same color combination as you!

AFRAID OF THE GRAY?

What is the worst thing that can happen? If you don't like it, you can always go back to coloring it again. You will never know what beautiful colors you have hidden under the dye unless you give it a try!

WHAT IS YOUR UNIQUE COLOR COMBINATION?

Cheyenne: My hair is red, blonde, gold, and white, with silver sparkles."

Jan: "I have white hair with tiny strands of charcoal mixed in. In the back I have dark brown and charcoal gray hidden underneath."

Trudy: "My hair is a combination of white, gray, charcoal, and brown."

Dianne: "My hair is white, gray, and black coffee."

Beth: "I have platinum hair, with a mixture of silver, gray, and white. In the back I have a small brown streak hidden underneath."

Deb: "I have white, silver, platinum, gray, and black hair."

Becky: "My hair is 75 percent snow-white, 10 percent shiny silver, 5 percent platinum, and 10 percent black."

Melissa: "I have light gray and white hair, with a chunk of dark brown at the nape."

Viv: "My hair is silver with strands of dark gray scattered throughout."

Bettina: "I am dubbed Silver Siren. My hair has many shades of gray and white."

Kay: "My hair is white and gray with a few black strands hidden underneath."

Dulcy: "My hair is light gray, white, and light brown."

Kathy: "I have white, silver, gray, and black hair."

Terri: "I have salt and pepper hair with a silver halo around my face."

Arlene: "My hair is a mixture of white, light brown, dark brown, very dark brown, auburn, and a few gold strands mixed in."

Jade: "My hair is beige-y platinum."

Linda: "My hair is calico! My color combination is silver, red, brown, and black."

Lynn: "I call my hair color silver maple! It is white, silver, platinum, blonde, dark blonde, light brown, and medium ash brown."

Barbara: "My hair is silver on top and brown underneath."

Nancy: "I have silver and pewter hair on top and around my face, with dark brown at the nape, and white at my right temple."

Raija: "I have white, platinum, and gray hair."

Dawn: "My hair is platinum. It's a mixture of very light gray, medium gray, and dark silvery gray."

Jodi: "My hair looks like cinnamon sugar! I have an assortment of browns mixed with white, and chunks of white in the front."

Gigi: "I have mainly white and platinum hair with strands of dark gray, gold, and strawberry-blonde mixed in."

Aqua: "My hair color is pewter, with silver strands mixed in."

Carmen: "My hair is platinum, white, and silver, with various strands of black, red, blonde, and brown."

Cathy: "My hair color is a mixture of browns, grays, gold, and black."

DH: "My hair is white on the top and front, and black in the back underneath."

gray8 color combo's

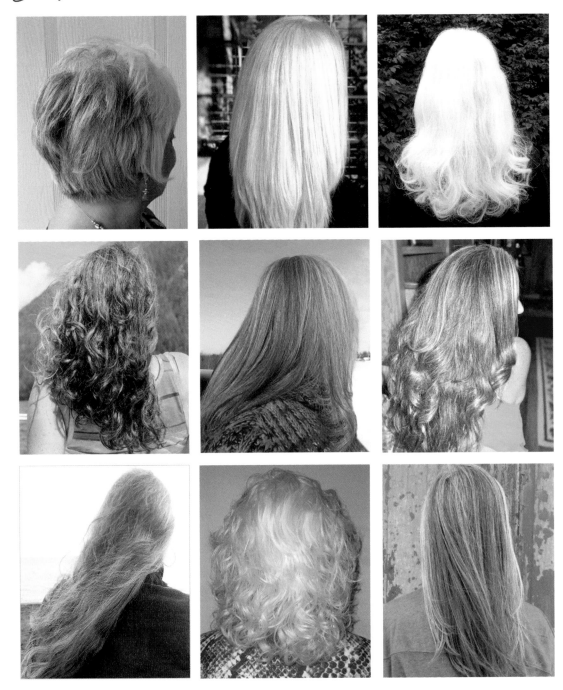

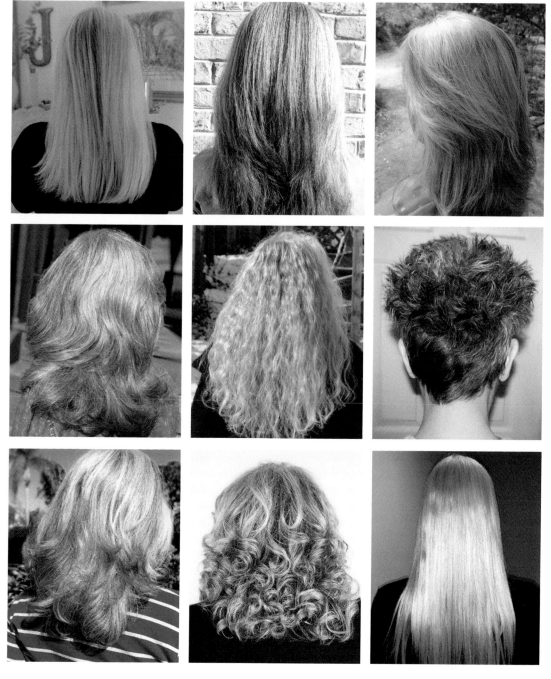

ditching the dye

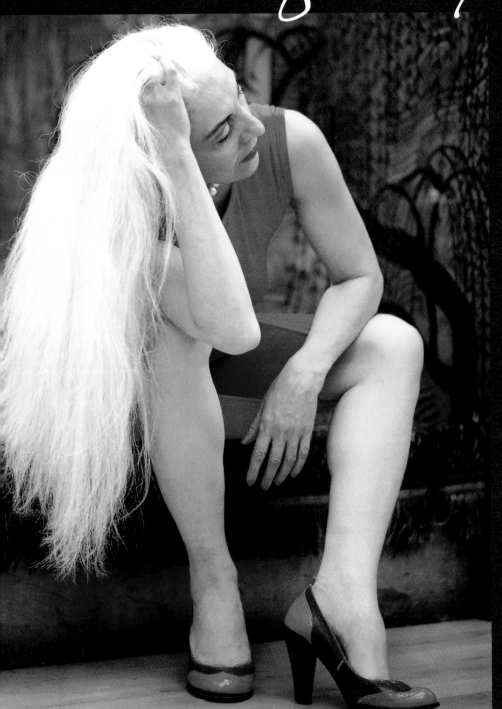

the long & short of it

When you decide to go gray it's definitely a big change, and takes some getting used to. Throw in cutting your long hair short, well... that could definitely put you on overload status! Especially if you are not used to short hair! Now, all of a sudden, you are faced with two transitions; going gray, and a short haircut! Throw in a bad haircut—well, we won't even go there! A gray8 place to start in the beginning stages of going gray is to first wrap your head around the transition process. Once you do that, if you decide to cut, you will be ready for that second transition. How do you know if you should cut or not? Simply ask yourself if you would wear the same short haircut with dyed hair. If the answer is no, don't cut! Cutting your hair will not make your hair grow any faster. You just have to decide if you want one inch roots with long hair, or one inch roots with short hair! Cutting will however expedite your transition.

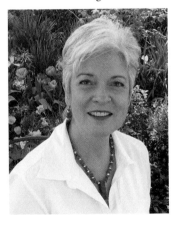

YOU control the length of your pixie by the amount of grow-out you have prior to the cut. Envision yourself after a pixie cut. Will you be transitioned? Will you still have dark ends? Would another month make you feel more comfortable? If you already wear your hair short, you may find that cutting it shorter; no big deal. In fact you may even consider a buzz cut. Sometimes it's hard not to snip, snip, snip away at the dye! The wash-and-wear and low maintenance of a pixie can certainly be very gratifying.

If you want to keep your length, by all means, keep it! An Ombre requires frequent tiny trims, and taking care of your dyed hair; not neglecting it. If you have long hair, and you are thinking about cutting, try taking baby steps instead; take a few inches off and "live with it." Once you become adjusted to your new look, take a few more inches off. Cutting a little at a time will give you complete control over the outcome. The profound look of an Ombre can be very empowering! Always remember; YOU control the length of your hair during your transition.

There is no right or wrong way to ROCK the SILVER! What may work for one person, may not work for you. Many women have chosen to keep their length, while just as many have gone for THE CUT! Whatever route (ROOT) you decide to take, remember... it is your head, your hair, your decision, your journey, and your life!

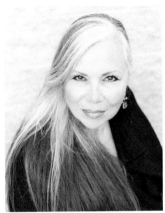

what's the best way 2 go gray?

Once you decide to "ditch the dye," your next step will be to determine how you want to transition. So we asked a few women, "What's the best way to go gray?" And this is what they had to say!

Benilda: "Buzz cut."

Kay: "Definitely cold turkey. Why defeat the purpose by applying color to your hair when the whole idea is to attain 'virgin hair?' When I stopped coloring, I wore my hair up, and used hats and other creative methods. Then, at the six month mark, I went to the hairdresser and had her cut my very long hair to shoulder-length."

Kama: "I went for the highlights, which helped me ease into the idea."

Nancy: "I went short with layers."

Diann: "Cold turkey worked for me. That said; patience isn't one of my better virtues, so I decided to cut my hair in order to speed up the process."

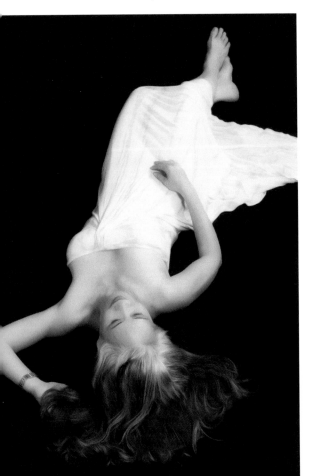

Kitty: "The best way for me was to go cold turkey. I took a deep breath and said, 'It's time.' I threw the hair color I had in the trash, found a support group via the Internet, kept trimming my hair, and rejoiced when the last bit of dye was cut off. Best is not always the easiest though, I think the easiest, would be to get a buzz cut and just let it grow."

Kathy: "For me, the most important thing was to look 'put together.' I would not have been able to feel that way, with dark dye on my hair when my natural hair was coming in so light. So I buzzed my hair off. Within six to eight weeks, I was sporting the JLC look. I could not have handled (even with a support group) two-toned hair, especially with it being so dark."

Helen: "I found a supportive group via the Internet in 2007. My then ten year old daughter had found her social consciousness and had donated her long blonde hair to 'Locks of Love,' along with several other girls in her class. So I followed her lead and just went cold turkey, but without the trims, and then had a big chop of nine inches to a bob cut!"

Kellie: "For me, it wasn't a choice; I had to go cold turkey because I found out I was allergic to the chemicals in hair dye. But, if I had a choice, I would not have changed a thing! I also intend to get a pixie cut. I'm excited about chopping it off since the ends are thin, dry, and frizzy. So I would suggest cold turkey, a cut, and a support group!"

Juanita: "It took several years to grow mine out, as I did not want to lose my past-waist-length hair."

Marjorie: "I stripped my hair, got highlights, went platinum blonde, and then got a pixie."

Becky: "Before the computer age, you just 'let it grow out' and dealt with it as best you could; it was called 'life.' Honestly, I don't know how some people go through the transition without some kind of support group!"

Shawn: "Cold turkey, but you need to do what's best for you!"

Rose: "I had my hair colored very light blonde using foils. I had been wearing it blonde for quite a while, but this shade was much lighter. Then, I had it cut short, not pixie short, but about two-inch layers. Every five weeks, I faithfully had it cut. In nine months, it was completely grown out, and it was absolutely painless."

Karin: "My hair is shoulder-length, and I have learned from experience that I don't like wearing my hair short. I stopped dyeing my hair, but didn't like the silver 'landing strip,' so I had highlights and lowlights put in to make the transition easier."

Kim: "My hair was finally growing out from a bad haircut, so there was no way I was going to go short again. I was looking for a change, and loved the way my sister's curly salt and pepper hair looked, so I quit cold turkey and wore a lot of pony tails."

Lindsey: "My stylist lightened the dark color a little bit each month. She also cut it in a stacked bob. As soon as I had about one-and-a-half inches of growth, I had it cut short. It only took a couple more months, and all the dye was gone."

Eloisa: "Cold turkey all the way, once I made the decision that chemicals did not belong on my head anymore."

Tara: "I went cold turkey. I don't like myself with short hair, so I compromised by growing out an inch and cutting off half an inch. I followed this routine until all the dye was gone."

Shaun: "I went cold turkey for four months. Then I had a family wedding to attend, and I didn't like the skunk stripe look, so I chopped it all off. I went from below-shoulder-length to a pixie cut. Boy, was that a shock to everyone, including me! Now it is finally growing out."

Debra: "Started off cold turkey, but then got lowlights at the four month mark to balance out the color. I snipped away like crazy at the old dye, especially during the first year, but never went shorter than just sitting on top of my shoulders."

Terri: "I went cold turkey. For me, it was easy; I just let Mother Nature take its course."

Sandy: "I didn't like the skunk stripe, so I got a pixie cut and grew it out. I thought this method was less painful than trying to cover it up."

Dulcy: "I did highlights twice. It was much easier for me to grow out highlights, than having a stark demarcation line. I wore the Ombre look for three years, as I have long hair. The highlights worked extremely well."

Heather: "I went for a pixie cut; I could not stand the wait."

Helen: "I had my hairdresser strip the dark dyed color from my hair. It was bleached twice and dyed an ash-blonde. My new gray roots matched the blonde color very closely, so the transition was made much easier. I have strong hair, which wasn't damaged by the process, and, for me, it wasn't about the chemical issue as much as making the transition as painless as possible. The bleach and blonde dye were applied to the lengths of my hair, not my scalp."

Bobi: "Cold turkey and a pixie cut for me."

Nicole: "I used hair coloring (root crayons) at first to disguise the skunk line. When my roots got longer, I did not like the stark difference between my roots and color. After seeing the new hair coming in healthier, I just wanted to be rid of the old-colored hair, so I got a pixie."

Rachel: "The first thing I did was to let just a gray streak grow in. After that, I decided to grow it all out. Then I had a few more highlights put in around my ears to ease the transition for when I pulled my hair back. Then cut it to shoulder-length."

Jen: "I went cold turkey, and I try to stay away from mirrors. I think it has been easier for me because I started with dyed blonde hair. I knew my transition would take longer because I refused to cut my hair shorter than shoulder-length."

Jayne: "I started coloring my hair at fifteen and continued coloring for 33 years! I wasn't brave enough to go cold turkey, so I added more and more blonde highlights to my dark brown hair until it was all blonde; then I let it grow out."

Laurel: "My complete transition took eight months. I began growing out a layered bob and kept trimming. Then, at seven months, I cut it into a short-shag. This got rid of all the dye except a fringe on my bangs. At eight months, I snipped off that fringe myself!"

Annette: "Cold turkey with pigtails."

Deb: "I quit cold turkey. I kept it short and powered through the many colors that worked their way out. Seriously thought about a buzz cut at one point but didn't do it. It took me about six months to transition."

Chris: "I started coloring my hair in my 20's, and continued until 60. No matter what color I used, within two weeks, it would turn a brassy orange from the Florida sun. I decided two years ago to stop coloring. I chopped off all my hair (as short as I could), without having to do a buzz cut, and just went from there. I just did it and held my head up high!"

Linda: "It took me about two years to transition. I had my hair cut to chin-length with layers and highlights. Once the layers grew out, I let it grow long. I love having healthy hair, and I don't have to worry about the roots showing anymore or putting chemicals on my head."

Julie: "It took me nine months to transition. I went from dark brown to dyed blonde hair with highlights. I kept my inverted bob for almost eight months and did regular trims every eight weeks. As my silver emerged further down my head, I used Roux Fanci-Full in True Steel, to help tone down the brassiness. In the eighth month, I took the scissors to my head and layered my hair to rid myself of most of the dye. Then four weeks later, I had the final (almost pixie) cut."

June: "I went cold turkey. It worked for me!"

Sheila: "I did not start off transitioning on purpose. I had been growing out my basically reddish hair, and my stylist had put in highlights/lowlights every four to five months for a couple of years. It made my hair look blonde, but really it was made up of five different colors, including the gray. Then my stylist left, and I couldn't find her. I was away throughout the summer, and still no luck finding a hairstylist. I felt that only 'she' knew my colors. At the end of August, I had searched the Internet and found all these beautiful ladies with wonderful gray hair. I had never even contemplated about letting my hair grow out gray, but I loved what I saw and hoped for the best! My hair was about five months in and not a lot of demarcation line, so I decided to roll with it."

Jo-Anne: "I decided for me, the best way to go gray was to get a full head of platinum highlights. I won't say the transition was completely painless, but it was not as bad as I thought it would be. Months four to eight were the worst! I wore a lot of hats."

Yvette: "It took me all of four months to transition. I kept cutting it every few weeks. I did not wear hats, scarves, or anything to cover my new silver color. I was proud of the growth."

Rebecca: "I highlighted and got a pixie cut for my transition."

Monica: "It took me eleven months to get to the point where I could not stand the two-toned look anymore and had my stylist give me a long pixie. I am letting it grow long now. Now I have healthy hair, and I don't have to worry about the roots showing or having to put chemicals on my head."

Janet: "My transition took twelve months. I went from just below shoulder-length hair, and gradually cut it shorter. I never went full pixie, but kept it at about chin-length with layers. I used Roux Fanci-Full Rinse in True Steel to help tone down the brassy dyed ends. While it didn't cover completely, it did help blend it in better."

Dawn: "Getting a pixie cut was a big help for me. I was able to transition in four months."

Shelly: "I made an appointment at the hairdresser's and had her bleach my hair to the lightest color blonde my hair would take. Then I let my hair grow for four months and had it cut into a pixie."

Peggy: "My personal preference for transitioning my colored hair to natural was to take the journey and make the most of it. I started with a consultation with my colorist to tell her my plan to discontinue regularly scheduled color appointments, and in turn, scheduled hair trims and shape-ups every six weeks. I used hair combs and headbands, but really, for me I just did a slow transition. To keep my length and similar shape, I had the length trimmed just slightly and the layers continually evened up."

Mary: "Cold turkey! I have mid-back length hair and decided not to cut. I sported the Ombre look and got regular trims."

skunk stripe

We have all heard the term "skunk stripe," but what exactly is it? It is the new growth of gray hair showing at the root line. In other words, our ROOTS! We disliked them when we colored our hair, and dislike them even more now; especially during the beginning stages of the grow-out. Today there are a variety of products on the market that can help camouflage the skunk stripe. ColorMark is a liquid hair color that can be applied with a soft-tip applicator, and washes out completely when you shampoo. Color Wow Root Cover Up, is a powder that you can apply with a brush to camouflage your roots; you will find lots of how-to videos on their website. Roux Fanci-Full Rinse is a temporary hair color rinse that refreshes, corrects, and tones the hair. There are also color-match dry shampoos that you can use to cover your roots. Highlights and lowlights are another option to help camouflage the demarcation line. Also there are plenty of hats, scarves, and stylish headbands! The word "skunk stripe" is not the most glamourous word out there, but one that is most likely here to stay!

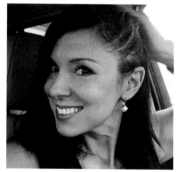
Misty Rogers: 1 month

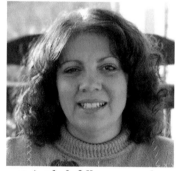
Lois Khalafalla: 1.5 months

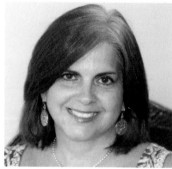
Debbie Smith: 2.5 months

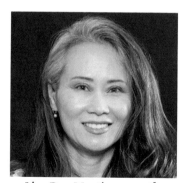
Lisa Dee-Martin: 3 months

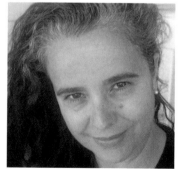
Eloisa Garoutte: 3.5 months

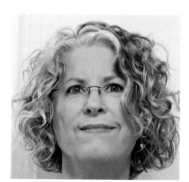
Noelle Smith: 4 months

buzz cut – transition

A buzz cut - transition, is an (all over the head), same-length, haircut. Cutting the hair in a uniform manner will insure an even growth pattern. A buzz cut - transition is quick, easy, and painless, and requires hair trimmers, new growth, confidence; and a lot of patience during the grow-out period! The length of your new growth will determine the length of your buzz cut. After a buzz cut, you will be fully transitioned. Now, all you have to do is sit back, and watch your graylicious hair unfold! Pip Bacon began her transition with a short pixie, but ended up cutting it all off to be an extra in a movie."

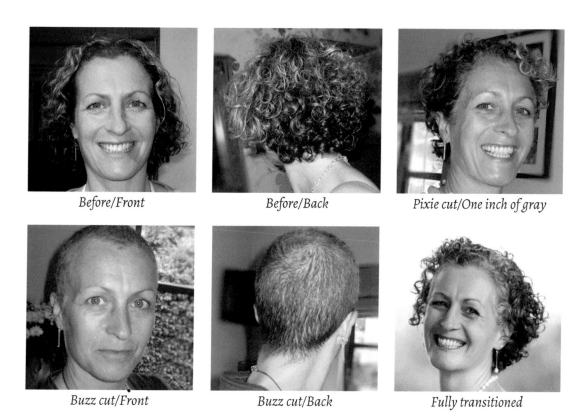

Before/Front   Before/Back   Pixie cut/One inch of gray

Buzz cut/Front   Buzz cut/Back   Fully transitioned

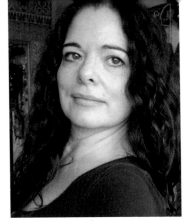

Before

cold turkey pixie cut — transition

A cold turkey pixie cut - transition, is when you decide to STOP coloring your hair cold turkey, and go for THE CUT, in order to expedite your transition. A pixie cut will vary in length, depending on the amount of grow-out you have, and your own personal comfort zone. As your natural hair grows in, you trim away at the dye, until you're no longer sporting a two-toned look. Sharon Rogers transitioned twice using the cold turkey pixie cut method.

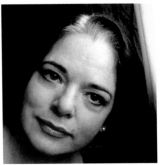

1 month

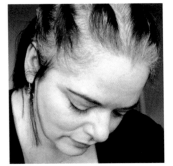

1.5 months

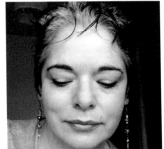

2 months

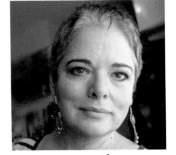

2.5 months

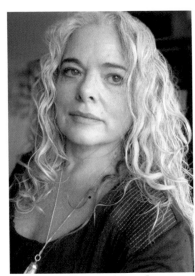

Fully transitioned

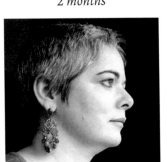

3 months

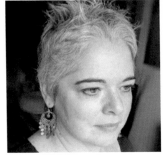

4 months

cold turkey length – transition

A cold turkey length - transition is when you decide to STOP coloring your hair cold turkey, and keep your length, while transitioning to graylicious hair. Amanda Meller (45), knew she didn't want to cut, and was determined to look her best while sporting two colors. She took care of both her dyed and silver hair by deep-conditioning often, and trimming when needed. She went from sporting the Ombre look, to AMAZING SILVER HAIR!

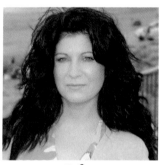

Before

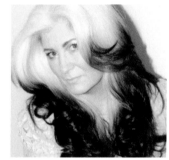

12 months

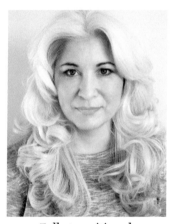

Fully transitioned:
2 years 4 months (front)

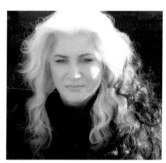

14 months

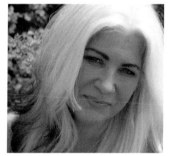

18 months

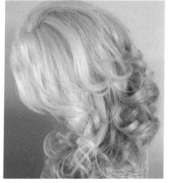

Fully transitioned:
2 years 4 months (back)

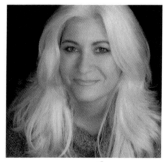

22 months

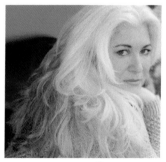

25 months

feathering – transition

The feathering technique is used to help camouflage the dreaded demarcation line between the new growth, and the dyed hair. For the feathering transition you continue to dye your already dyed hair, and have the stylist feather-it-in with your "new gray growth." This method will extend your transition time, but a gray8 option for someone who:

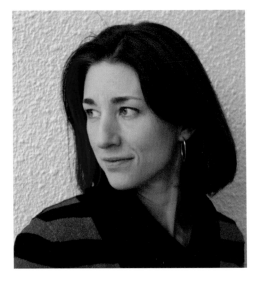

- Wants to keep their length

- Does not want to deal with the demarcation line

- Is not allergic to hair dye

- Does not want brassy ends

- Is in no hurry to transition

Emily (38) stopped dyeing her hair last spring, and has about five inches of uncolored hair. She decided early on, that she wanted to keep her length, but didn't want brassy ends, or the "forever" demarcation line. So she had her stylist color her "already dyed hair" and feather-it-in with the new gray hair. She had this procedure done twice during her transition. Emily also has a white streak that is the full length of her hair. She discovered a white patch several years ago; had the color bleached out, and wore her white streak while she continued coloring her hair. She also colored it magenta for a year.

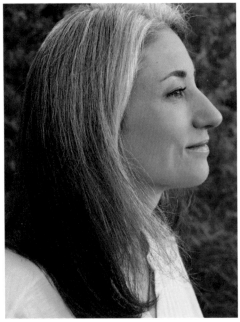

highlights/lowlights – transition

A highlights/lowlights transition is traditionally used to help camouflage the demarcation line between the new growth, and the dyed hair. Highlights lift color, and can be any shade, as long as it is lighter than your overall hair color. Lowlights add color, and can be any shade as long as it is darker than your overall hair color. Lowlights give depth to the hair strands. When getting highlights/lowlights, the foils should not be brought up to the scalp level to avoid touching the new growth. Start foils at the demarcation line, avoiding gray roots. If you add highlights/lowlights to the dyed hair only, you will NOT be adding to your transition time. If you add highlights/lowlights and include your new gray roots, you will need to start your transition over.

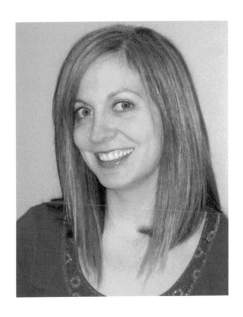

Dawn Hofstad

1 month
Blonde/Gray highlights/lowlights.

Dawn received both highlights and lowlights to help ease her transition. Professional Colorist Wendi Gossen explains, "I lifted Dawn's old color in a foil to a level 9 and toned it with 9B and 9V. I added a cool tone (level 5 Ash) to her hair that was left out." Please note: This recipe is listed as a courtesy for your hair care professional.

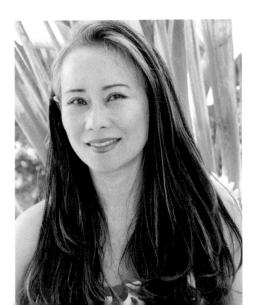

Lisa Dee-Martin

3 months
Blonde highlights

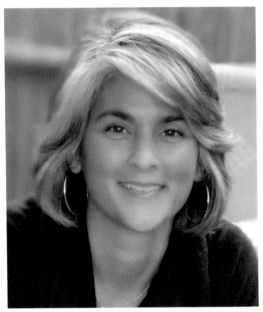

Monica Gallacher
5 months
Highlights/Lowlights

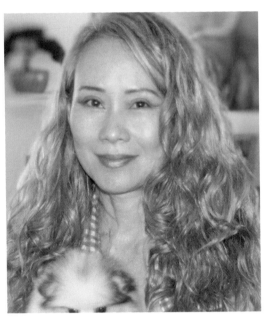

Lisa Dee-Martin
7 months
Gray highlights

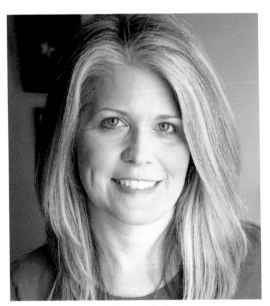

Cathy Meinke
7 months
Blonde highlights

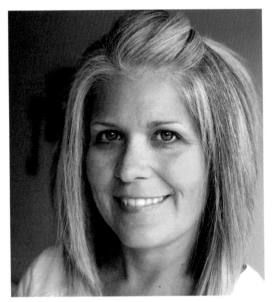

Cathy Meinke
10 months
Blonde highlights

Helen Smith went from dark to platinum, with two inches (4 months) of growth. Helen said, "I went from brown to blonde all in the same day after a very 'long day' at the salon." Helen's hair was in excellent condition prior to this procedure. Always consult with a hair care professional. If your stylist says no listen; you do not want to carry your hair home in a bag! (Helen's "after" picture was taken nine days after going platinum.)

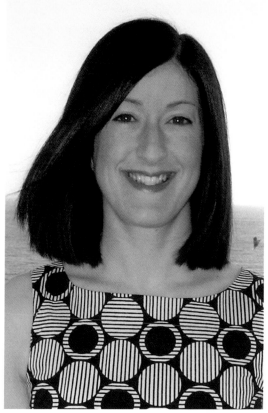

Helen Smith
Before

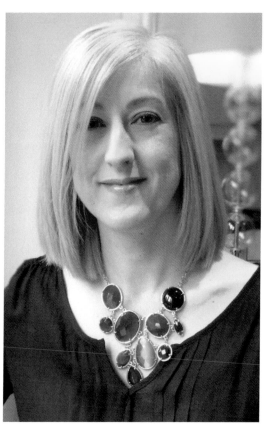

Helen Smith
4 months
Platinum highlights

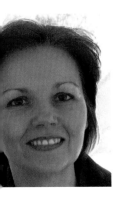
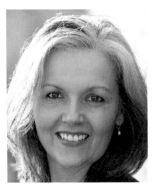
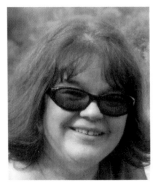
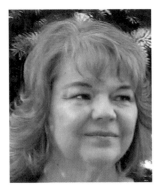

gray8
before & after
pictures

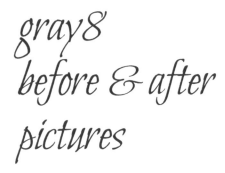
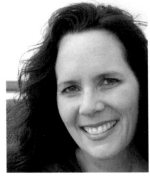
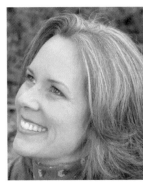

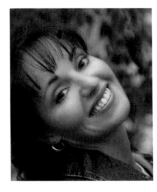
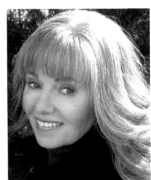

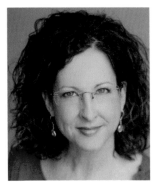
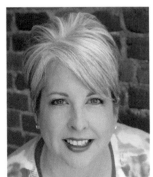

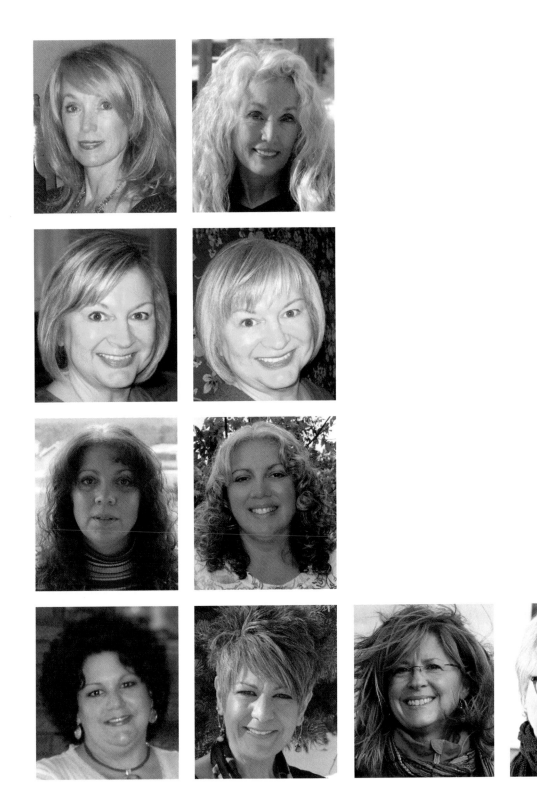

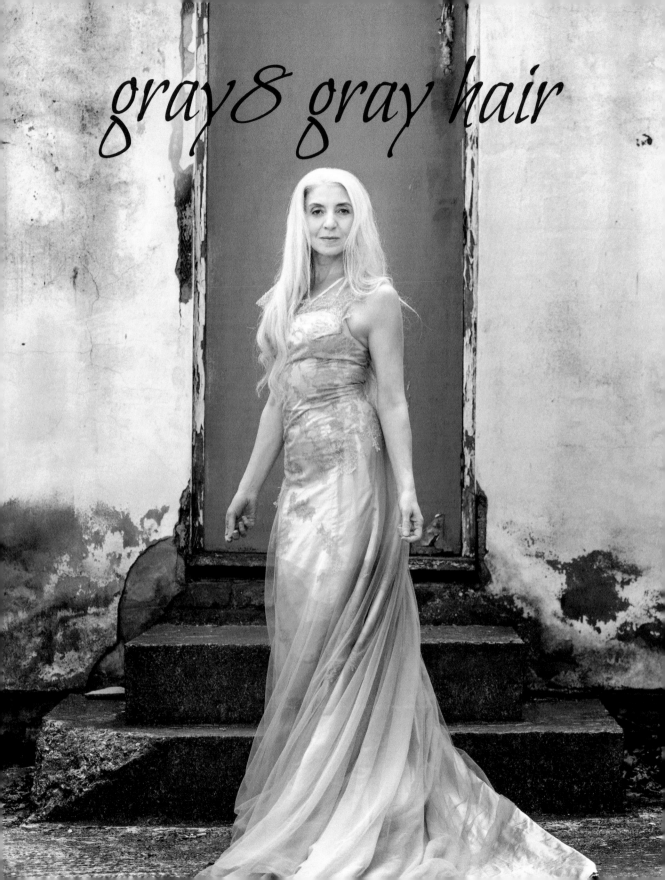

gray8 gray hair

10 gray8 reasons 2 go gray

Everyone has their own reasons for wanting to go gray, and GGG has a few more reasons to add to that list! You don't have to accept society's limited definition of beauty—we certainly don't!

1. A unique color of your own
2. Authenticity/Uniqueness
3. Being a role model/It's OK to go gray
4. Easy on the pocketbook
5. Elegance/Sexy/Graylicious
6. Freedom/Liberating
7. Free highlights and lowlights
8. Healthier hair
9. Less maintenance
10. Self-confidence

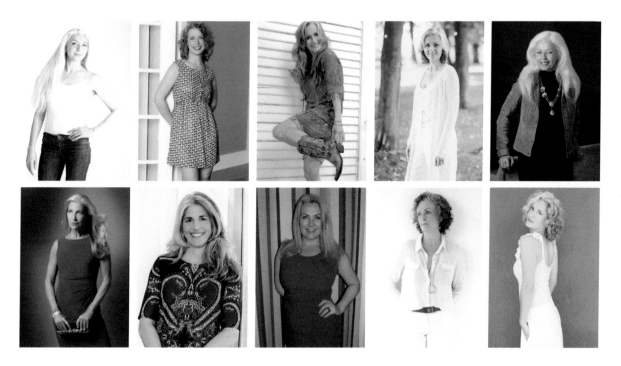

10 steps 2 gray8 silver hair

1. Stop over-cleansing! Shampoo twice a week and rinse with water in-between shampoos.
2. Use a clarifier or purple shampoo only when needed.
3. Air-dry your hair whenever possible. When using heat-styling tools use low setting, and heat protectant spray.
4. Do not apply oil to your hair before you use a flatiron; it will scorch your hair.
5. Keep hair nourished with oils, leave-in conditioners, and deep-conditioning treatments.
6. Use clear or white styling products.
7. After you apply makeup, lotions, etc. wash your hands before touching your hair.
8. Keep hair trimmed and styled.
9. A few styling options: finger-comb, wide-toothed comb, boar bristle brush, and wood bristle brush.
10. Sleep on a satin or silk pillowcase to prevent frizz and breakage.

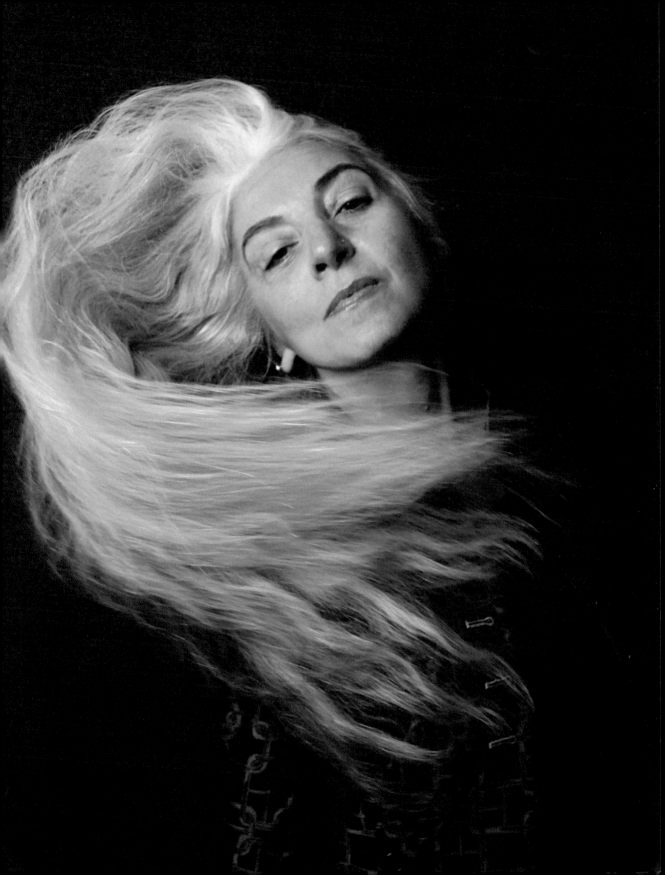

10 gray8 products 4 shine

1. AG Hair The Oil Extra Virgin Argan Miracle Smoothing Oil
2. Alberto VO5 Conditioning Hairdressing for Gray/White/Silver/Blonde Hair
3. Aveda Brilliant Spray-On Shine
4. Carols Daughter Monoi Oil Sacred Strengthening Serum
5. Coconut Oil
6. L'Oréal Mythic Oil
7. MOROCCANOIL Treatment Light
8. Paul Mitchell MARULAOIL Rare Oil Treatment Light
9. Pureology Colour Stylist Cuticle Polisher
10. Redken Outshine 01 Anti Frizz Polishing Milk

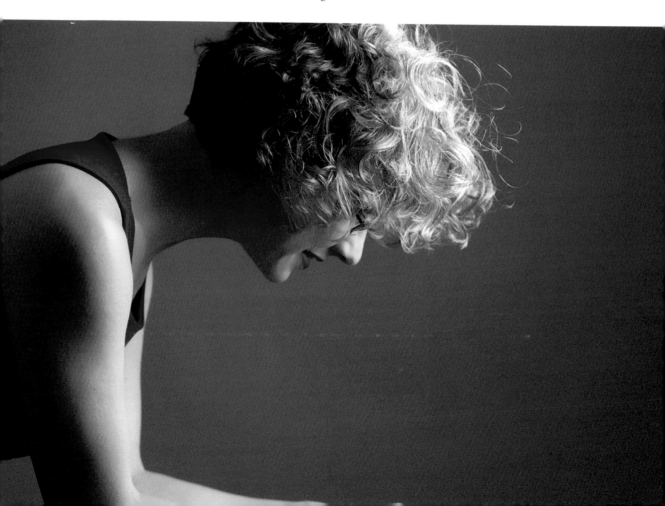

10 gray8 products 4 style

1. AG Hair Moisture & Shine Fast Food Leave On Condition
2. Aveda Brilliant Retexturing Gel
3. Curly Hair Solutions Curl Keeper
4. DevaCurl Light Defining Gel
5. Jessicurl Spiralicious Styling Gel
6. L'Oréal SLEEK IT Iron Straight Heatspray (protects up to 450 degrees)
7. Matrix Biolage Styling Curl Defining Elixir
8. MopTop Curly Hair Custard
9. Pureology Perfect 4 Platinum Miracle Filler
10. Redkin Extreme Anti-Snap and Redkin Frizz Dismiss

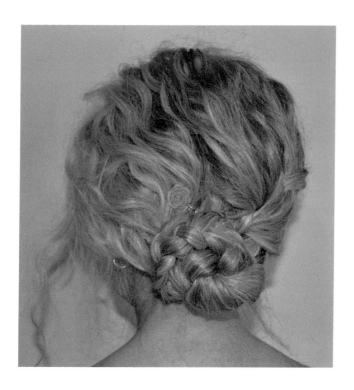

10 gray8 ways to wash long silver hair

How someone washes their hair, isn't something we normally talk about; I mean how hard can it be? Right? For years I washed my hair in the exact same way; I piled it up on top of my head, and scrubbed it, like some kind of crazed woman on a mission, never once giving it a second thought. I hurriedly washed my hair each morning for work, blasted it with the blow-dryer, and then when flatirons came along, I added that into my hair care regime as well. Finding hair on the bathroom floor and in my brush was the norm. It wasn't until years later, that I realized the damage I was doing to my hair. So... let's take a look at how others wash their hair.

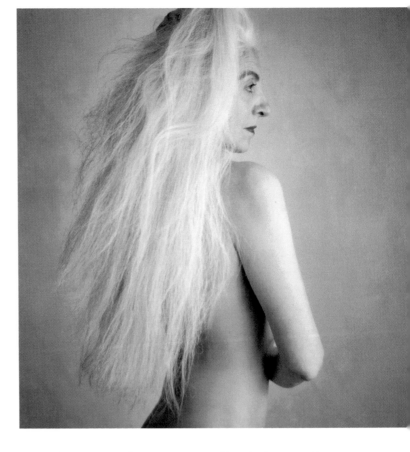

Beth: "First I get my bra-length wavy hair wet. Then I concentrate on using shampoo on my scalp only, and let it slide down to my ends, and rinse. Since I have long hair, I do not want the friction of rubbing my hair together, to cause damage. I very seldom lather up twice. When I use conditioner, I concentrate on my ends instead of my scalp and seldom rinse it all out."

Debra: "I have straight, almost bra-length hair. First I wet my hair in the shower. Then I dilute a small amount of shampoo in a cup of water. I pour it over my hair and gently massage my scalp with my finger-tips to cleanse, (I do not pile my hair on the top of my head). Then I rinse thoroughly. To condition: I use my cup again, but this time I add conditioner to it. Again I dilute the conditioner in a cup of water, and pour it over my hair; ear level down. I use a wide-toothed comb in the shower to work the conditioner through my hair and to remove any tangles. I let the conditioner sit (while I finish washing), then rinse my hair again. I wrap my freshly washed hair in a towel, to absorb the excess water, (but do not rub my hair with the towel). I remove the towel, and use my fingers to remove any tangles before using my wide-toothed comb."

Dulcy: "To cleanse my below waist-length hair I use baby shampoo. I stand in the shower, keeping my hair down my back (less tangles). I wet my hair and cleanse my scalp using my finger-tips, using a short back and forth motion, and then rinse. I use conditioner (only on my ends) then rinse again. After I shower I wrap my hair in a micro-fiber towel for about five minutes to remove extra moisture. Then I apply a detangle spray, and use a wide-toothed comb. I let my hair air-dry or use a fan to dry my hair. My long hair dries in ten to fifteen minutes. Once my hair is fully dry I smooth out my curls with a boar-bristle brush and sometimes wear a bun (no elastic) for about five minutes to further naturally smooth my curly hair."

Gloria (Gigi): "My routine is very simple. I always wash my curly/wavy hair in the shower, but only about every third day, (when I wore my hair short, I had to wash it every day). First, I wet my hair, add a little shampoo, and then massage my scalp with my finger-tips, and rinse. Sometimes I like to switch out what products I use, as my hair responds better that way. Then I add a small amount of conditioner, and work it through my hair with my finger-tips and rinse again. I attribute my ability to grow my hair fast, and as long as I have; due to using Pro-V Pantene Beautiful Lengths products. When I get out of the shower, I wrap my (just above bra-length) hair in a Norwex Hair Turban. I leave it on for five to ten minutes, to absorb the majority of the water in my hair. Then I use Sami Fat Hair Thickening Cream. I put a small amount on my finger-tips and then work it through my hair; from the roots to tips. This product makes my fine hair feel, and look, so much thicker. Then I use my fingers to comb my hair, and let it air-dry. If I want my hair to be smoother, I gently use a blow-dryer with a large round-brush, and use warm/cool air. Afterwards, I use my curling-brush for a quick roll-up; using a shot of warm air, and then a shot of cool air, and unroll. That gives me a nice soft curl."

Jan: "I wet my shoulder-length, wavy hair, in cool water (not cold), as I believe it helps maintain my natural oils and adds shine. I apply DevaCurl No-Poo, (while my hair hangs straight), and use both hands to apply it liberally throughout my hair. I use my finger-tips on both hands to massage my scalp, using a front to back motion (not back and forth), to avoid friction and tangles. Then I rinse my hair and apply conditioner (ears down). I use my finger-tips or "Wet Brush" to comb the conditioner through my hair and remove tangles. At the end of my shower I rinse my hair thoroughly. Afterwards I put a tee-shirt on my shoulders and use the tee-shirt to gently squeeze my ends. Then I apply a small amount of Redkin Extreme Anti-Snap Leave-In, and DevaCurl Supercream. If I want extra volume, sometimes I use DevaCurl B' Leave-In. Then I scrunch my hair to add wave and that's it!"

Janice: "I use WEN Cleansing Conditioner. I wet my hair, and run a handful of WEN through my hair, all the way down my straight bra-length hair. I add water and cleanse my scalp with my finger-tips, and rinse. I apply a second handful and work that through my hair in the same way. After I add a little water, I put it on my head, (if it will stay there) until I finish my shower, then rinse. I then apply a little leave-in conditioner and either finger-comb it or use a wide-toothed comb on my hair. I use a tee-shirt for a towel."

Kathy: "I have bra-length curly hair and use Carol's Daughter Milk Co-Wash to cleanse my hair. I massage my scalp with my finger-tips in a back and forth motion, and let the shampoo run through the rest of my hair. After I rinse my hair, I use a conditioner and gently use a wide-toothed comb to distribute it through my hair. I hold a section of hair in one hand, and hold my comb in the other. I start at the bottom and work my way up, doing a little at a time. Since I have curly hair, I don't want to comb my hair once it's dry. Sometimes I plop my hair, or just let it hang down and let it air-dry."

Kay: "I wash my bra-length hair three times a week in the shower, using shampoos that offer protection against damage. I massage my scalp with my finger-tips using a back and forth motion, and let the shampoo run down my hair, rather than pulling my hair up. Afterwards, I use conditioner only on the ends of my hair, I let it sit a minute, then rinse. Once out of the shower, I apply a leave-in treatment (mostly on the ends), then I apply a heat protector, as I use a blow-dryer to remove excess wetness, then I let the balance air-dry. Once my hair is completely dry, I use a heated brush mainly at the crown for lift, and carefully pull some of the curl/waves out. I also take Biotin."

Kitty: "I normally wash my almost waist-length hair, in the morning. I begin by using lukewarm water, and let it run over my hair for several minutes. Then I use conditioner to cleanse my scalp. I massage my scalp with my finger-tips in a small circular motion. I rinse again, and pour a large amount of conditioner into the palm of my hand, and work it into my hair. Then I squish it up, toward my scalp, for at least a minute; this really brings out the curl. Then I rinse again using the same squishing method. I gently run my fingers through the length of my hair to remove loose hairs, and then squish it again. I wrap it all up in a cotton tee-shirt, and let the curls fall loose. To add lift to the crown, I put in about six clips, and let my hair air-dry."

Marni: "First I saturate my bra-length hair. Once I apply shampoo, I use my finger-tips to gently massage my scalp and hair. I rinse my hair while it hangs straight, and then rinse again, with my hair flipped. I follow the same procedure with my conditioner. After the final rinse, I add a leave-in conditioner and Jessicurl Rockin Ringlets. Then I gently squeeze my hair with a tee-shirt, and tie it around my hair (like a cap). I leave it on about twenty minutes, then scrunch my hair, and let it air-dry. If I'm in a hurry, I blow-dry my hair on low/warm heat with a huge diffuser. I use my fingers to comb my curly hair."

10 gray8 mistakes

1. Cutting long hair too short—too soon.
2. Using a henna, semi, or demi-permanent dye to camouflage roots; it won't rinse out.
3. Letting a stylist add highlights/lowlights to your gray roots.
4. Turning your dyed hair orange with do-it-yourself hair lightening concoctions.
5. Drying your hair out by over using brightening shampoos, and whitening products.
6. Scorching your hair with heat styling tools. Use a temperature control with heat protectant.
7. Getting highlights after you complete your transition; they will look yellow with your natural hair.
8. Looking for gray hair under the dye; it's not there.
9. Allowing naysayers to dictate how "you" should wear "your" hair.
10. Announcing your decision to go gray on social media; it will solicit naysayers.

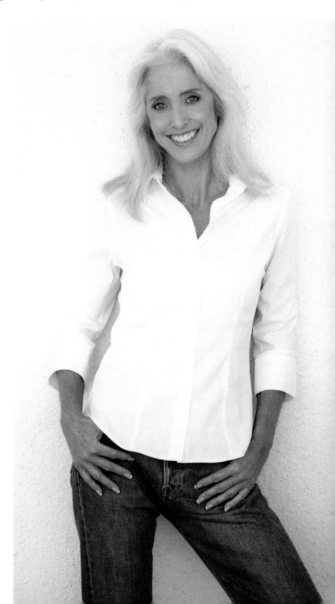

10 do's & don'ts 4 hair loss

Hair loss is something I am no expert on, nor want to become an expert on; but unfortunately have experienced it firsthand. There are various reasons for hair loss: thyroid, hair dye, styling products, heat-styling-tools, hormones, aging, illness, medication, diet, genetics, stress, and who knows what else I forgot to mention! I have had hair loss twice, so the first thing I did was get my thyroid checked. My thyroid came back fine, so the exact reason? Who knows! But thankfully my hair came back. WHEW!

The second time I had hair loss, I made a doctor's appointment seven days out. I learned from the first time, that in order to be taken seriously, I was going to collect the hair that I lost each day, and put it in a separate baggie. When I showed it to my doctor, she said, "WOW, you really are losing a lot of hair!" Okay—now I was really worried! But, because my doctor had seen the hair loss firsthand, I was taken seriously, and I didn't get the famous comment, "It's normal to lose up to 100 hairs a day."

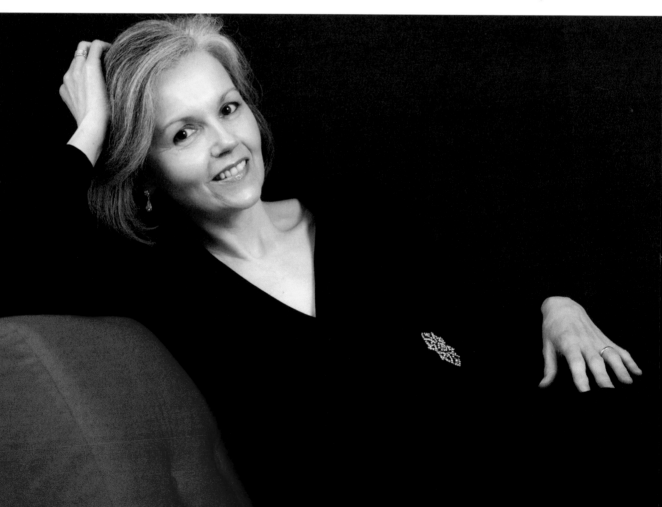

The doctor drew blood to check my thyroid, and asked about my medications, diet, medical history, etc., and put me on a hair vitamin. She also suggested that I cut my hair (to get the weight off) and avoid pulling it back in a pony to alleviate some of the stress put on the hair. At my follow-up appointment, I was told my thyroid results came back fine, so now what? Stress? Menopause? Most likely both LOL! But how can you not be stressed when you are losing your hair?

Several months later my hair stopped falling out; talk about a stressful situation! Going through hair loss can be devastating, so check with your physician and find out why YOU are losing your hair! Meanwhile, here are a few hair loss tips I have picked up along the way.

DO'S & DON'TS

1. Do see your doctor and get your thyroid checked.
2. Don't use heat-styling-tools during hair loss.
3. Do let your hair air-dry.
4. Don't use a brush when your hair is wet; your hair is more fragile.
5. Do eat nutritional meals! Diet can have a direct effect on your hair.
6. Don't over-cleanse or wash your hair aggressively; be gentle!
7. Do massage your scalp with your finger-tips or head massager to stimulate circulation.
8. Don't forget to take your hair vitamins and get plenty of rest.
9. Do use a satin pillowcase or place a satin scarf over your pillow to avoid breakage.
10. Don't let it stress you out!

10 contributors & solutions 4 yellowing hair

10 CONTRIBUTORS 4 YELLOWING HAIR

1. Chlorine
2. Foods high in carotene
3. Health
4. Heat-styling-tools, i.e., flatiron, blow-dryer, etc.
5. Medication
6. Pollution
7. Smoking
8. Styling Products
9. Sun
10. Well water/Mineral deposits

10 SOLUTIONS 4 YELLOWING HAIR - PURPLE SHAMPOO

1. AG Hair Sterling Silver Toning Shampoo
2. Aveda Blue Malva Shampoo
3. Clairol Shimmer Lights Shampoo
4. Jhirmack Distinctions Silver Plus Ageless Shampoo
5. Joico Color Endure Violet Shampoo
6. Matrix Total Results So Silver Shampoo
7. Paul Mitchell Platinum Blonde Shampoo
8. Pro:Voke Touch of Silver Brightening Shampoo
9. Redkin Blonde Idol Custom-Tone Conditioner Violet
10. White Hot Hair Brilliant Shampoo

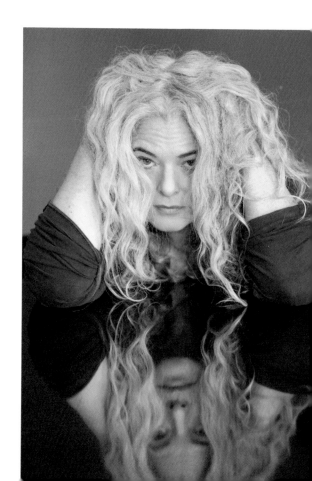

10 SOLUTIONS 4 YELLOWING HAIR - CLARIFIERS

1. Carol's Daughter Rosemary Mint Clarifying Conditioner
2. Ion Clarifying Shampoo
3. Joico K-Pak Clarifying Shampoo
4. Kenra Clarifying Shampoo
5. MOROCCANOIL Clarifying Shampoo
6. Neutrogena Anti-Residue Shampoo
7. Paul Mitchell Clarifying Shampoo Three
8. Pureology Purifying Shampoo (zero sulfates)
9. Redkin Hair Cleansing Cream Shampoo
10. Suave Daily Clarifying Shampoo

BAKING SODA (SODIUM BICARBONATE) CLARIFIER

Although baking soda is a unique cleaning agent/clarifier, it is also abrasive, as it contains crystalline grains, which can break, weaken, damage, and dry out your hair. High-alkali products, like baking soda, open up the hair cuticle so that your hair absorbs water. When this happens, your hair may weaken. To counteract and close the cuticle, a vinegar and water rinse should be used. Never use straight vinegar on your hair. Make sure you read everything there is to know about this natural home remedy, as it can damage your hair.

NEWNESS 2 GRAYLICIOUS HAIR & PURPLE SHAMPOO

Finding the right hair product is no easy task. Your favorite shampoo is not necessarily going to be someone else's favorite. I look at hair products in the same way as I do makeup and skincare. If you stop at the makeup counter and try on a new product, you may need to stop at a few more, before you find the right one that works best for you. I spent years managing cosmetic departments, so I know firsthand that women with the same skin types may require different solutions, based on their individual needs. Hair is pretty much the same way, gain product knowledge, and be your own best judge in what products work best for you!

Use a purple shampoo to counteract yellowing in your hair. Violet (a secondary color) is directly opposite of yellow (a primary color) on the color wheel; when mixed together, they cancel each other out. Note: Not all purple shampoos are created equal, usually the deeper the purple, the higher the concentration. Blue shampoo works in the same way. Blue is opposite of orange on the color wheel, so if you have orange and brassy-tones in your hair, you will want to use a blue shampoo.

When we first turn silver, all we can think about is keeping our silver hair, shiny, bright, and white! But what happens with this new found excitement is that we start over using products, only to dry out our graylicious hair! Just like when we put detergent in the washer, if a little works, imagine what using a little more might do! But purple shampoo is not going to give you white hair! It will only brighten what you already have, and help remove yellowing. Over use of purple shampoos and clarifiers can eventually dry out your hair. You should not be using a purple shampoo everytime you wash your hair. Under normal circumstances, once a week should be sufficient (less often during the winter months), especially if you already have dry hair. But, (there is always a but!), if you are dealing with hard/well water, you are also dealing with mineral deposits that can cause yellowing to your hair. To counteract this, you may need to use a purple shampoo or a clarifier more often, so condition, condition, condition—to keep dryness to a minimum!

Another note about purple shampoo: I have heard from women with very white hair (myself included) that their hair actually darkened over time due to build-up from purple shampoo, taking months to rectify. The build-up was so gradual and did not take on a blue or purple-ish tint. The hair only became a darker shade of gray, so they never related the two. Once they "cut back" on the amount of purple shampoo they were using, or, in some cases, stopped completely, their white hair made its debut once again! So, whereas one person can use a purple shampoo once or twice a week, someone else may only be able to use it once a month or, in some cases, not at all. If you have very white hair and this happens to you, try using a very small amount of purple shampoo mixed-in with your regular sulfate-free shampoo, or use a clarifying shampoo once a month instead. If you have white hair, do not let purple shampoo sit on your hair for any length of time, in order to avoid a gray tint. If you have porous hair, try using a lilac shampoo instead of a dark purple one, or switch to a clarifier. If you have a darker shade of gray, and your hair is taking on a dull look, you may also want to consider the possibility that you may have a build-up, caused by overuse of purple shampoo.

gray8 gray hair

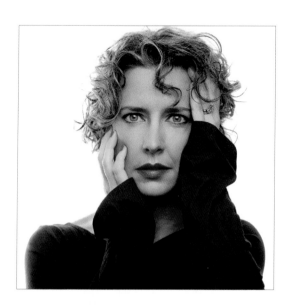

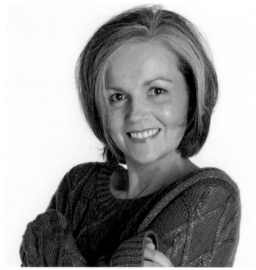

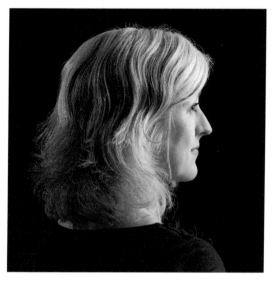

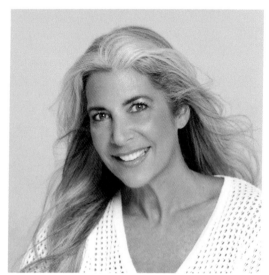

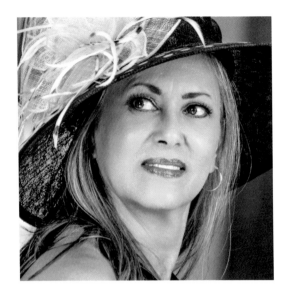

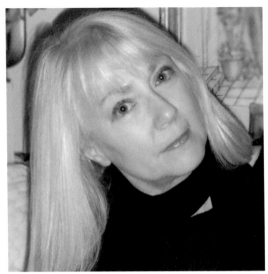

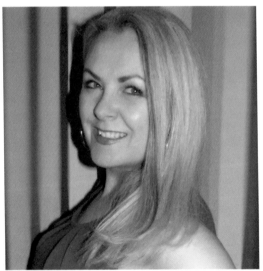

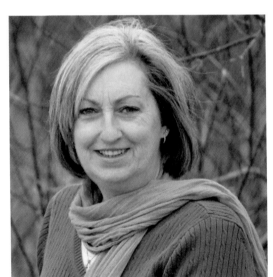

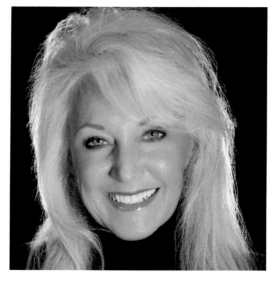

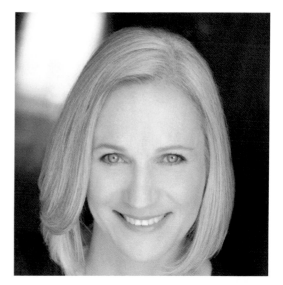

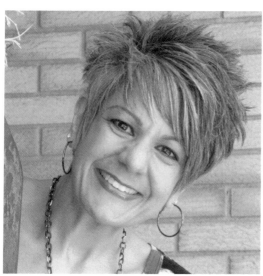

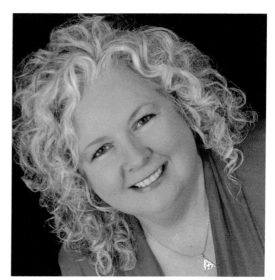

gray8 curly hair advice

BY CURLY HAIR SPECIALIST SCOTT MUSGRAVE

MagiCurl Blog http://www.scottmusgravehair.com/
Author and Founder of Curly Hair Artistry http://www.curlyhairartistry.com/

SILICONES - CONES - SILLY CONES

Silicones, cones, or what some like to refer to as "silly cones," are found in many hair products, conditioners, and styling products. They can build-up on the hair shaft, and prevent proper hydration that is required to keep hair elastic, soft, and in a state of growth. Silicones are a form of plastic that accumulates on the hair shaft. Build-up can cause the hair to swell and eventually cause breakage, creating thousands of different hair lengths all over the head. You end up with uncontrollable frizz, and a halo effect of loose hairs. To avoid this, your hair products should say: silicone-free, sulfate-free, and paraben-free.

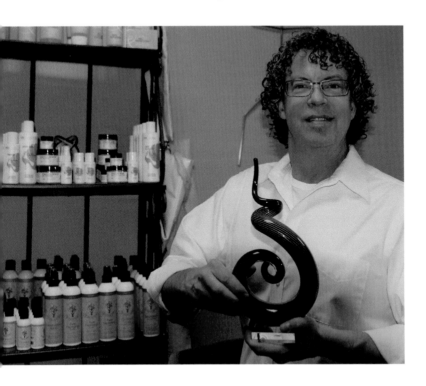

When you stop using silicone-based products, your hair starts a journey of healing. It is so exciting and truly magical (MagiCurl) to see your hair return back in much better condition! Products ending in cone, conol, and xane should be avoided.

SILICONES

- Amodimethicone
- Behenoxy Dimethicone
- Bisaminopropyl Dimethicone
- Cetearyl Methicone
- Cetyl Dimethicone
- Cyclomethicone
- Cyclopentasiloxane

- Dimethicone
- Dimethiconol
- Phenyl trimethicone
- Polydimethylsiloxane/PDMS
- Stearoxy Dimethicone
- Stearyl Dimethicone

SODIUM LAURYL SULFATES & PARABENS

For a healthy scalp, it is best to avoid sulfates and parabens whenever possible. These ingredients can be found in shampoos and other products. Sulfates are used to create suds, but can be abrasive and dry-out the hair, causing breakage.

CURLY HAIR MESSAGE

Curly hair does not need to be fixed, it needs to be embraced! I only work with your curls as they are, and refuse to straighten them, comb them, or use a towel on them, and, NO flat-ironing allowed in my studio!

Two years ago, I started a group to help other stylists learn the art of working with curly hair, without being brand specific. We now have over a 100 stylists (from all over the world), that meet every day to discuss hair color, products, cutting, and business management. We meet twice a year in salons, hosting approximately 30 stylists from locations such as: Australia, Brazil, Canada, UK, Newfoundland and all over the USA.

what a gray8 question

question: *"I have been in transition for two months and got a very short haircut. I'm not sure I like my gray hair. What should I do?"*

answer: Two months of growth will not give you a clear picture as to how your hair will look once you complete your transition. Give it time; as your hair grows, different shades will unfold. I believe Mother Nature always gets it right. It could very well be the "short haircut" that you don't like. The beginning stages of going gray are sometimes difficult, but the rewards are plentiful. You owe it to yourself to see this through. You will need a lot of patience when it comes to growing out gray hair! Meanwhile, sit back and enjoy your graylicious ride.

question: *"Would you recommend a color corrector to remove the dyed color from my hair? I am anxious to see what my gray hair looks like underneath."*

answer: Unfortunately, you will not find any gray hair under the hair dye; that ship has sailed. Your hair shaft has been altered. In order to have gray hair you will need to grow it out and not color the gray roots.

question: *"I want to go gray but really want to avoid the skunk stripe. I was told I could use a semi-permanent dye on my roots. What do you think?"*

answer: Do not add color to your roots. Because once you grow out your permanent dye, you will need to go back, and grow out your semi-permanent dye. See the word permanent? Bottom line, if you don't see a skunk stripe, or dye free hair at the root line, you are not transitioning.

question: *"My gray hair is darker in the back, is that normal?"*

answer: Yes. It is very common to have a darker shade of gray in the back. Sometimes it is hidden under a lighter shade of gray, so you may not realize that others have it too.

question: *"I am three months along in my transition and I'm concerned that my hair will completely wash me out, what do you think?"*

answer: It usually takes several months to get a good idea of what your hair will look like; your hair will change as it grows. Right now, it's too early to tell, and it may appear lighter next to the freshly dyed hair. If you feel washed out once you complete your transition, you can always add color back in with a small amount of makeup, along with some colorful accessories and wardrobe pieces.

question: *"I was told I shouldn't use a flatiron with gray hair. Why not? My hair is too unruly without it!"*

answer: Yes, you can still use a flatiron with gray hair! BUT, choosing the right flatiron is important and can literally "make or break" your hair. No doubt, ironing your hair can cause yellowing and breakage, so look for a flatiron with high quality plates and a temperature control and use the lowest temperature available. After reading hundreds of posts, darker shades of gray seem to do better with

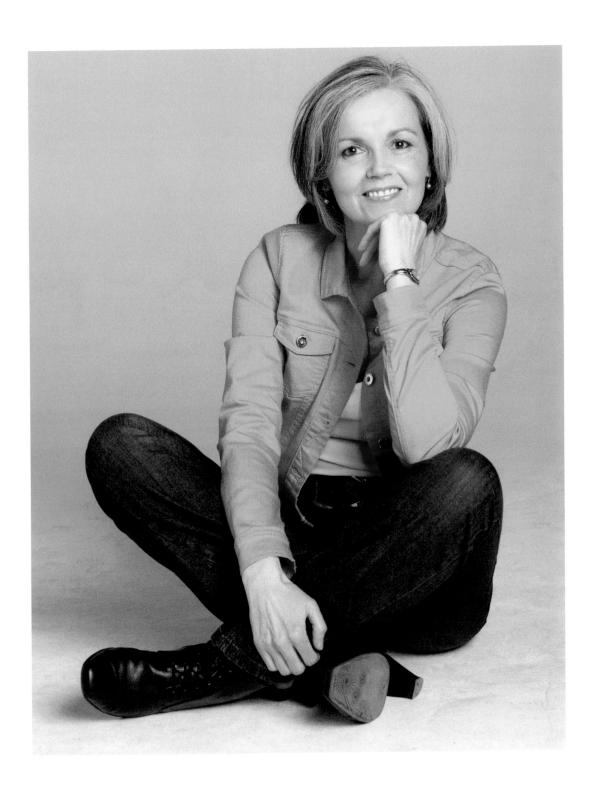

a flatiron than white hair. Those with white hair, find that their hair yellows, and, scorches easily, showing every flaw. Remember to apply a heat protectant prior to ironing your hair.

question: *"How do I go gray gracefully with gray roots?"*

answer: Roots are roots; there is nothing graceful about them! Keeping your hair groomed and being your best self, will take you far when it comes to growing out your gray hair gracefully! There are many products on the market that can help camouflage the beginning stages of going gray! You can get pretty creative with hair crayons, headbands, hats, and scarves. Having a bad hair day? Take the attention off your hair and wear your best outfit, put a little makeup on, and bring out the widest, sparkly, headband you can find! If all else fails, hold a cute baby! That will definitely take the attention off of you!

question: *"Can lighting affect the color of my gray hair?"*

answer: Yes! Gray hair is transparent, so it reflects light and surrounding colors. Move over a foot or change the color of the top you have on, and your hair will suddenly take on another hue. Your hair will reflect differently indoors verses outdoors. Outdoor lighting will give you a truer picture as to how your hair actually looks.

question: *"Why do some people think gray hair equals old?"*

answer: Because in the past, the only place we saw gray hair was on little old gray-haired ladies. Gray hair has been associated with old-age for a very long time! Think about it—even the ancient Egyptians created henna to color their hair! Old traditions are hard to break! As little girls, we grew-up with commercials telling us, that in order to look young, we must cover the gray. But in all reality, we now know, looking young has little to do with hair color. In the future, how society looks at gray hair will depend on us. Educating them is a gray8 place to start. Once they see more of us out there, they will start seeing things in a different light.

question: *"Why is my scalp pink?"*

answer: When we dyed our hair, we also dyed our scalp along with it. If you feel you are seeing too much pink and it bothers you, use TOPPIK hair building fibers to cover. HSN also sells a hair fill & color kit by Signature Club A.

question: *"How long will it take me to transition?"*

answer: Hair grows approximately half-an-inch a month. How long it takes you to transition will depend solely on the method used. Cutting your hair short will be the quickest method at four to six months.

question: *"Why does hair turn gray?"*

answer: Going gray, for most part, is unavoidable. As we age, our pigment (color) cells start to die off, resulting in transparent hair or what we refer to as variations of gray. Genetics, lifestyle, health, and environment also play a role. Many experience seeing their first gray hairs as early as in their teens, while others are in their 20's, 30's, and, older. There is a lot of gray out there! We just don't see it under all that hair dye!

question: *"I want to go gray, but my children are totally against it, and tell me that I will look like grandma. What should I do?"*

answer: Children learn what we teach them. If you are okay with it, they will be okay with it too. We teach our children to accept their own differences, so why not teach them to accept ours as well? Not everyone will have the privilege to grow old; educate them that it's okay.

question: *"I have almost black hair and have decided to go gray. I don't have a problem with gray hair; my problem is with short hair. Currently my hair is mid-back. I need to find a way to transition without a pixie, any suggestions?"*

answer: Many women grow out their natural hair color without sacrificing length. You can easily rock an Ombre, by keeping your dyed ends trimmed, and conditioning often. Another option would be the feathering transition, you can read more about this in chapter two.

question: *"I ran into an old friend, and she said she didn't recognize me. Do you think it's because of my gray hair?"*

answer: NO! Not everything is going to be about your gray hair. Once you have settled into your new look, you will understand what I mean. It is very normal for someone not to recognize another person, especially if you're not seeing them on a regular basis. Even a pair of sunglasses, haircut, weight gain, beard, etc., can throw someone off. Your brain collects a picture image of someone, and it stays that way until it's been updated. Think of it this way; remember your high school classmates? If your image has not been updated, you remember them as they were back then, not as they are today. Give your brain time to re-boot! After a while, you will be looking at your old photos with colored hair, thinking, "That doesn't look like me!"

question: *"I have dark hair and want platinum highlights, but my stylist said no! Is getting platinum highlights that big of a deal?"*

answer: Trust the advice of your stylist! The condition of your hair most likely will not be able to tolerate the strong chemicals needed to lift it to a platinum level. You do not want dry, brittle, crunchy, straw-like hair. Nor do you want it falling out on you! Dark hair may take a couple visits to the salon, in order to lift it slowly. Start with blonde highlights and deep-condition often. Once your hair is in better condition, check back with your stylist to see if it's possible to go lighter.

question: *"I am 27. I want to gray, but everyone says I'm too young. What do you think?"*

answer: If you have gray hair, obviously you're not too young to go gray; you're already gray! Now, to decide if you want to show the world or not! Even if you don't have gray hair, what could be healthier than having 100 percent natural dye-free hair? I think being young adds an exciting twist to gray hair, and, no doubt, you will look striking! Besides, we need women like you to change the way society thinks about gray hair and beauty. Growing out gray hair can be a challenge, especially during the beginning stages, but once your transition is complete, you will not be disappointed! You will find, that keeping your hair in great condition with a current hair style always "trumps" whatever hair color you might have. Ultimately, the only opinion that matters is YOURS. If YOU want to go gray; go gray!

question: *"How do I protect my gray hair when I go swimming?"*

answer: Try wetting your hair down with clean tap water or distilled water first. Wet hair will not absorb chlorine as quickly as dry hair. Use a swimming cap and add a little conditioner so your swimming cap goes on easily. Remove chlorine afterwards with a chlorine-removal shampoo.

question: *"Why should I go gray? My dyed hair makes me feel young!"*

answer: If your dyed hair makes you feel young, then by all means keep it! BUT, it doesn't mean you look young; especially if you are still using a dark color. As an Esthetician I know that your face is the true tell-all, not your hair! Bottom line: All that matters is how YOU feel about YOUR hair! Gray hair is not for everyone. It's your head, your hair, and your decision! But if you're the slightest bit curious, why not give it a try? What's the worst that can happen? If you don't like it, you can always go back to the BOTTLE! Not everyone that goes gray stays gray, but many end up transitioning for the second time.

question: *"I'm only a few months into my transition; do you have some witty comebacks for all those unsolicited comments I seem to be getting on coloring advice?"*

answer: How we learn to interpret comments is very important to our self-esteem. For example if someone said to me, "I would never go gray," that would not bother me... I would never go purple. It doesn't mean I don't like purple hair, it means that I don't like purple hair on ME. Not everyone is going to like the same things as you do, and that's okay! When someone makes a comment always ask yourself first, if THEIR opinion really matters. Meanwhile I posted this question to GGG, and here is what a few of the women had to say:

- "I simply smile and say thanks, but I love my gray hair!"

- "Going gray is popular right now!"

- "I developed an allergy to the dye."

- "My hair quit falling out a ton when I quit coloring!"

- "I tell them my gray hair became resistant to hair color."

- "Dye irritates and burns my scalp."

- "I'm incorporating a healthy lifestyle."

- "When someone I don't know makes a comment about my gray hair, I tell them it was between ditching the dye, or ditching my husband, and that usually ends the conversation!"

question: *"I am having a hard time finding a stylist who supports me during my transition; I am getting a little frustrated. Can you help me?"*

answer: First, don't get frustrated, this has nothing to do with you personally; coloring hair is a big part of what they do! When you sit down, let your stylist know up front that you love your gray hair, and have no intentions of coloring. A good stylist will embrace your decision. If she is not onboard and makes flip remarks, find another stylist!

question: *"My stylist said I can't go gray because my pink undertones will wash me out. Is that true?"*

answer: Actually, I know a lot about pink undertones from first-hand experience, (I have them too)! Your pink undertones will actually give you some added color. Your pink undertones are going to be there, no matter what color your hair is. Yellow skin correctors, such as Clinique's Superprimer Face Primers and Clinique's Redness Solutions, Mineral Pressed Powder, can help camouflage the pink. Silver hair can lighten and brighten your face, minimizing facial lines, etc. If you are feeling a bit washed-out, adding a little color back in, is as easy as one, two, three! Take three minutes and apply a little mascara, blush, and lipstick. You will not be disappointed!

question: *"I have just started the growing-out process. Will I need to change my makeup and wardrobe colors?"*

answer: You will undoubtedly want to make some changes to your makeup colors, but, for the most part, they will be minor. There are three colors that will determine your makeup colors: skin color, hair color, and eye color. (It's also important to know your skin's undertones.) If you have fair skin and white hair, you will definitely want to balance things out by wearing makeup. But it doesn't mean you need to wear a LOT of makeup; neutral colors in eye makeup and soft subtle colors will work perfectly fine! I recommend you stop at the cosmetics counter and talk to the Beauty Advisor/Consultant. She can do a makeover on you and suggest some gray8 colors for you! For wardrobe, unless you need an excuse to buy all new clothes, try adding in some bright-colored scarves and colored jewelry, to accentuate your already existing wardrobe. Look at the different undertones in a color, example; yellow-orange and red-orange. I love red-orange with my skin tone, but yellow-orange; not so much! Also if you have white hair, your hair may appear yellow next to a bright white. So take a second look at whites, beiges, and yellow-creams. Yellow-green, red-brown and rust, most likely will bite the dust depending on your skin tone. But, before you discard anything, wait until you are fully transitioned! Jewel-tone colors look gray8 with gray hair! When in doubt wear a colorful scarf! If you want to know your perfect colors, consider a color analysis.

question: *"I have a ten year old picture of myself displayed on my mantle (with dyed hair). A friend of mine noticed it, and commented that I have really changed. Do you think it's my gray hair?"*

answer: In all reality people do change during a ten year span; it's called aging. We can't blame ten years of physical changes on hair color alone; time to put out a current picture!

question: *"What should you do when your husband or significant other is not on board with your decision to go gray? I am sure I am not the only woman who has felt this resistance. I have always worn long dark hair, but recently got a short pixie. Do you have any suggestions?"*

answer: Wow, that's a toughie, although I know it happens. My guess is, that he is used to seeing you with "long dark hair," not a "short pixie with gray roots." So that's a lot to take in all at once. You will need to reassure him it's not going to stay that way, and he will indeed get used to the new you! My theory in life is this: If it's important to you, make it important to him. A sit-down heart-to-heart conversation makes it important. Express your concerns and find out his, especially if you are experiencing some type of an allergic reaction to the hair dye. I am sure your health comes first and foremost in his eyes. I posted this question on GGG, and here is what a few of the women had to say:

Gaia: "My hubby is taking it pretty much like yours, he is not supportive, to say the least. I'm only twelve weeks in, so I hope to hang in there. When I told my husband about my decision to go gray, he said 'Why? It will only make you look older,' yet his hair is all gray! Men can go gray, and women can't?"

Mary: "My husband was skeptical about my decision to go gray (I'm six months in). I let him know that gray is just like any other color that I've played around with throughout the years. I've also asked him to withhold his opinion until I've finished growing it out completely. Then once I have transitioned, if it doesn't look good, I can always change it back (doubtful)! But, to his credit, even though he has his doubts, he's still going with the flow!"

Elizabeth: "My husband wasn't on board about me going gray, but now finds it rather sexy and says the color suits me perfectly!"

Eloisa: "Just hang in there, when all is said and done you will look radiant, and he will be on board. My husband was very supportive, but men are very visual and he had a hard time imagining how my hair was going to look after I was transitioned. So I showed him lots of pictures online of women rocking the silver. Some men also don't like the idea of having their wives go gray because it reminds them of their own age and mortality. Now that I am all done, he loves it!"

Aqua: "I did this for me! I realize that not everyone can be fully confident in their going gray journey, but you need to prepare yourself for the ups and downs and get through it, because the end result will be amazing!"

Joan: "Perhaps his negative take is due to your going natural and cutting off all your long hair at the same time. I would suggest that you tell him you will be growing your hair long again!"

Tracie: "My husband is not happy or supportive about me going gray. This is about his insecurities, not mine. In the meantime, during the yucky grow-out, I've been experimenting with different hairstyles, new tops, and pretty scarves!"

Michelle: "I'm sorry you've encountered resistance. I can understand how your husband's lack of enthusiasm might affect your confidence in making the decision to grow out your gray. The truth is, the transition is quite a drastic change when going from dark hair to gray—I know first-hand. Your husband may just need time to adjust to the change in your appearance. A few years back, my husband shaved his goatee and mustache that he'd been sporting for years, and it completely changed his look. I had always associated that facial hair with him, so when he was suddenly without it, I often felt like I was looking at a stranger, and I told him as much! Although I supported his decision to shave, it didn't mean that the change to his appearance didn't affect me. I think maybe that's the case with your husband, he might just need time to process the change you're making until he becomes accustomed to seeing you. And, while you may not need his approval, you probably respect his opinion and take it into consideration in many aspects of your life. That doesn't mean, however, that you're a slave to your partner's wishes; it means you're normal. Of course, you want the man you love to continue to find you attractive. Of course you experience trepidation when he expresses uncertainty about your choice in changing his established image of you. The bottom line is, your husband loves you and wants you to be happy! Yes, it's your hair, but like everything else in a committed relationship, you're in this together, and you deserve the same support you offer him in the choices he makes."

question: *"Will I still look sexy with gray hair?"*

answer: I believe looking and feeling sexy, involves a little more than a person's hair color; but I could be totally wrong about that! LOL! Looking sexy is a mindset! If you were attractive and sexy with colored hair, no doubt you will still be attractive and sexy with gray hair! Hair color does not determine if a person looks sexy or not, it's the total package that counts!

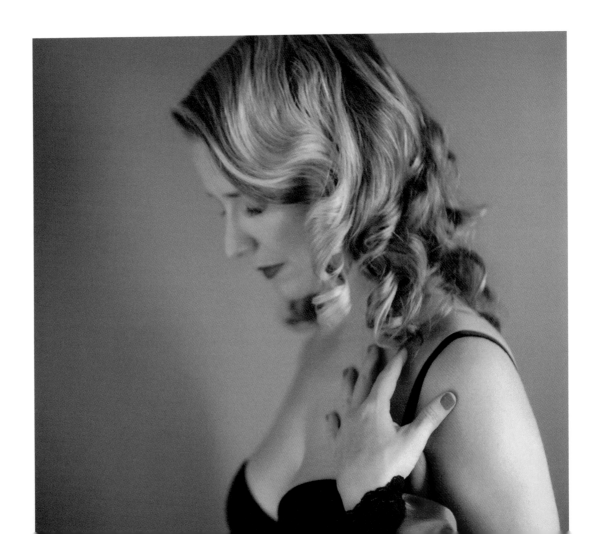

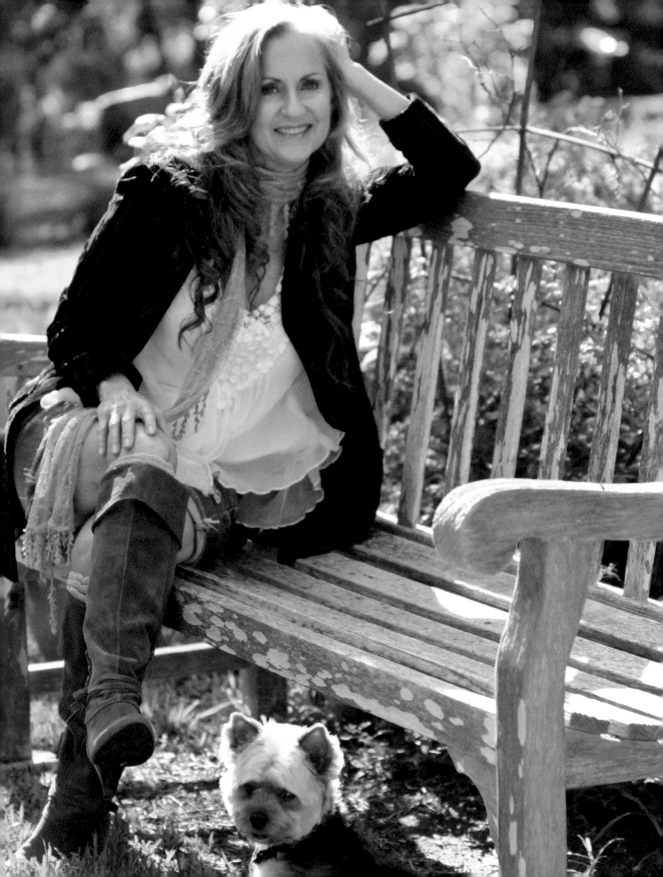

50 gray8
going gray stories

Alex B.
Age 55
London, England

I am a model who does commercial and editorial work. I am also an art model who poses for painters and sculptors.

Originally from Italy, I have lived in the UK for many years. I attended a university in London and for several years had a career in the academic field. Though I go back to Italy to visit my family frequently, London is my adopted city, my true home. I have been married and have one adult child.

I am dance-trained, in both ballet and contemporary, and occasionally still perform. I am very active and a regular gym-goer. I particularly like swimming. I also practice Sleek Technique; it's based on ballet, with lots of ballet barre work. It keeps me very supple. I love spas and sometimes treat myself to a spa day. I love water, steam rooms, and massage treatments.

I wear my grey hair very long—below my waist. My grey hair has helped me in my modeling career,

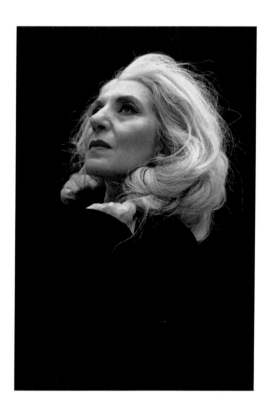

as it has given me a very distinctive look. I have been featured as a hair model for a range of hair products targeted at women and men with grey hair.

I began to go grey when I was 24, but I coloured my hair until the age of 40, when I finally decided to go "au naturel." I was tired of dyeing my hair on almost a weekly basis. On a whim, I got a pixie while traveling in Slovakia soon after my 40th birthday, and I came back feeling lighter and happier.

Within weeks, my hair was salt and pepper. It looked gorgeous. I kept it short for quite a while, but I am blessed with thick hair that grows very quickly, so I soon began to experiment with length. I found a very understanding, supportive hairstylist, who loved my hair colour and was able to advise me on its care.

Meanwhile, after attending a casting back in 2005, I was catapulted into modeling. At first, I was cautious and wore my hair in a bob in order to be suitable for commercial work (which is quite conservative in terms of look), but then I decided to grow my hair very long. This helped in transitioning to editorial work, as it gave me a quirky look.

I believe grey is a colour and should be accepted as such. It is not necessarily a sign of old age. Many women in their 30's have grey hair. I also believe that it should be up to each individual to decide whether they want to colour or not. I also do not think that colouring is wrong; it should be a choice. I would hate to be prescriptive.

GRAY8 TIPS & TECHNIQUES

I am a swimmer, so I protect my hair with a swimming cap and use an anti-chlorine shampoo soon after my swim. I use purple shampoo on a regular basis and condition my hair at least twice a week. I regularly use organic hair products and insist on heat protection when using tongues and hair dryers. As a model, I am always negotiating with hairstylists about the degree of heat of straighteners and such, especially since I once had my hair burnt yellow by a less-than-savvy hairstylist, and I did not relish it. It took ages to get rid of the yellow ends.

I have my hair trimmed every three weeks or so. Otherwise, I really do very little to maintain it. I will probably cut it very short again by the time I am 60. I sometimes get really tired of having long hair, as it tends to get in the way. To achieve a nice wavy look, I sometimes braid my hair before going to bed and, in the morning, I have lovely waves. It never fails, especially if your hair is still slightly damp when you plait it!

Photo credit: Natalia Lipchanskaya

Amanda Ball

Age 42

Tennessee

I am married, and have been working in administration at a research hospital, for the past ten years. My passion for horses, traveling, and Spain run deep, I am bilingual, with a husband from Barcelona, where I lived for nearly five years. We met in the Pyrenees Mountains in Andorra, a small country between France and Spain. I have been blessed with many life-changing travel adventures, job titles, and character roles, but now let me tell you about my most recent silver journey.

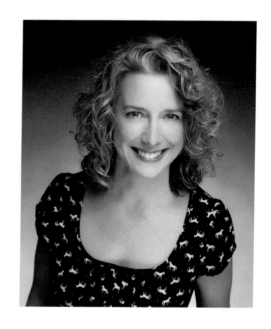

Having gray hair is uncommon among younger women in the South, including conservative Memphis. I remember seeing my first gray hairs in my early 20's, but just ignored them. Then, fifteen years later, when I was around the age of 35, ignoring them became impossible.

Before I ever found a web site or Facebook page about support for going gray, two women inspired me. One was a lady in one of my equine groups, maybe ten years older than I, who grew her hair color out and looked fabulous. The other; was a stranger in a picture, about 30-years-old, from an "O Magazine" article, "The Age Defiers." I still have her beautiful photo with the article pinned to my bulletin board. These two ladies' examples pulled my internal trigger, causing no backfire!

During this endeavor, here's what happened on the outside of my head. The coloring of my hair lasted for about four years, and, during this time, I went through various phases of screwed-up colors. Not knowing where to go for help, I first tried very expensive salons, but was still unhappy with the outcome. I wanted my ash-brown color back, and all the experts were leaving my hair with a red tone, no matter what I insisted! I ended up at a local hair school, where they turned it bright red, and then had to strip it, which left it carrot orange. With my hair fried, I took matters into my own hands and found a less harsh chemical color and did it myself at home. Kelley Van Gogh was the product, but I soon grew tired of the mess, cost, and dependence on the product.

Meanwhile, on the inside of my head, I decided I did not want to be coloring my hair monthly for the next 25 years, so I thought why not give gray a try while I still had a youthful face? I could always go back to coloring if it didn't work. I had a romantic picture of myself as a wise, long-gray-haired woman, authentic and comfortable with herself and with the horses and people around her. What did I have to hide from? What would it be like to step into this new hair role, and how would it transform me, my perspective, and the environment around me? I could be a trailblazer of sorts, a silver hair blazer, albeit a terrified one! Ridiculous ego-chatter drama kept flashing mental pictures of me being shunned by people at work, being asked to retire or leave early, getting fired, and causing societal shock waves in my small circle of friends and family. In other words, I was experiencing real "mental mayhem!"

On cue, via my equestrian friend, I ended up down in Senatobia, Mississippi, in a small local salon about 45 miles south of Memphis, where I met her stylist. She would help me transition with color, highlights, or lowlights—but once I got started, I decided to go cold turkey with no coloring. I then cut my hair in stages, from all the way down my back, to shoulder length, to a sort of bob cut, to finally getting sick of the color and insisting that she chop it all off! She didn't want to, but I was totally comfortable. "I never thought we'd have it THIS short!" she exclaimed.

While growing it out, I wanted to hide my hair. I was nervous and ashamed, so I kept it pulled back, flattened and discreet. There were, of course, some adverse reactions and feedback. But they were tremendously fewer than I imagined, and the compliments far outweighed the negative comments. It wasn't until the shortest phase that people really started noticing that my hair was silver and tri-colored. I started getting a lot of compliments, at work, in the airport, on the street—many folks, (mostly women), asking if I colored my hair that way. In the end, it was a self-esteem booster for me because my hair did look and feel fabulous. It had not been that healthy or dye-free in years.

After completion, I have two regrets: the reticence, shame, and loneliness I felt from listening to the "mayhem mind babble" during the transition, as well as a lack of documenting my progress with photos. I also realized that while covering my gray with dyes, I hid behind the faux color and its intrinsic toxic chemicals, in the habitual monotony of stifling social standards and unhealthiness. But I can now say that, via this voyage, I have found authenticity, empowerment, uninhibitedness, health, and strengths unfathomable before the completion of my change. Still today, my gray hair is a quiet power that I grow into as it continues to grow out. My hair is getting longer now, and I love it! Indeed, gray hair is a power, offering wisdom that women grow into as it grows out.

After the final personal struggle and physical appearance adjustment, I found flourishing online support communities for going gray. I was SO elated to know and connect with other women like myself. It was a self-esteem booster extraordinaire! I am so grateful, via these virtual groups, to have constant affirmation of confidence and companionship with my silver journey today.

Growing out my gray hair was like writing a daily permission slip for me to be myself, and I was determined to be myself! Thank you to each and every woman who chooses this adventure. Ultimately, we are all connected.

GRAY8 TIPS & TECHNIQUES

I like trying out new products, and like using ones that are free of parabens, and too many unpronounceable chemicals. My current favorite silver shampoo is ShiKai Color Reflect Platinum Shampoo. I wash my hair every other day and use shampoo with the ShiKai only once or twice a week, and use

Nature's Gate Shampoo most of the time. After shampooing, I apply any of Nature's Gate Conditioners; my current favorite flavor is chamomile. For my curly hair, I use Aveda Be Curly Style-Prep; it works best when my hair is damp. When I use hairspray, it is Aveda Brilliant. I use medium hold with chamomile. Since my hair is pretty thin, I blow-dry my hair as little as possible. I use the dryer more in the winter time, than any other time of the year, but only because I cannot stand to be cold!

My advice to you is to find the online groups! Take a proverbial sledge hammer to the mental mayhem babble that goes on within you. If that doesn't work, do a quick visualization of a handy laser gun and shoot that sucker the minute she starts up! Stop and breathe. Tea or coffee with a supportive friend helps, too. Take care of yourself on the inside and the outside. In the end it's all the same reciprocating care.

Photo credit: Guillermo Umbria

Anne Thomas Gerhardt
Age 49
Ohio

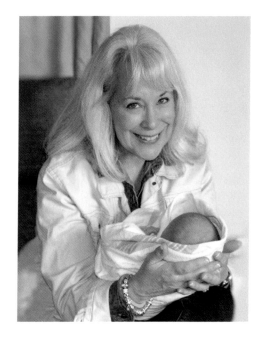

"It's a Family Affair."

My earliest memory of my grandma Murphy was her warm hug and beautiful white hair. My mother has the same warmth and stunning white hair. Lucky for me, I also inherited the lovely hair. But I wasn't always appreciative, of the premature silver locks.

My experiment with hair color started when I was in my teens, with a product called "Sun-In." As the gray hairs started to sprout, highlights helped hide the gray. By my late 20's, I was all in with all-over hair color. I had light ash-brown hair with highlights that would quickly turn orange in the sun. It didn't take long before eventually retouching the skunk stripe became a bi-monthly chore, and I became increasingly uncomfortable with the burning sensation on my scalp.

Seven years ago, when I was 42, I looked at myself in the mirror and asked, "Why are you putting yourself through this nasty process and adding more chemicals to your body?" I knew from my mom and grandma exactly what to expect if I went with my natural hair, so that didn't make me nervous. I just did not know "how" to transition. Only one book was available at the time, which mostly gave examples of women after the transition. The only support I had was from an understanding hairdresser and an older sister, who were both going to go through this with me.

I cut my hair into a short bob, and had regular highlights and lowlights put in, until I was mostly blonde. Gradually, we weaned off the highlights and, at nine months in, I was totally dye-free. By fourteen months, I was done and have never regretted the change. There have been a few insensitive comments, but the good compliments I received from strangers (about my lovely hair); far out-numbered any negative remarks I ever received!

My grandma and mom inspired not only me, but my beautiful sisters as well, with their confidence and ability to age gracefully. All three of us are proud to be SILVER SISTERS!

GRAY8 TIPS & TECHNIQUES

Getting highlights helped camouflage the demarcation line during my transition. I would also suggest NOT using a flatiron, especially if you have white hair. The heat can scorch your hair and turn it yellow. Many styling products have wax derivatives, which, combined with the heat can discolor white and silver hair. My favorite hair product is Lifeshine Oil by White Hot Hair. I use a blow-dryer on low-heat or a fan to dry my hair. I occasionally use hot rollers or a hot-air-brush for smoothness and curl.

Becky Baldry Hansing
Age 67
Texas

I am mom to four children and grandma to eight wonderful grandkids. We raised our children in Wisconsin, but moved to Texas in order to be close to our family (they are my heartbeat). I am a Midwestern girl, born and raised, but have lived all over the USA with the love of my life, Larry. We have been married 47 years. I work as an apartment manager during the day, and a couple of evenings a week, I work at an ice cream kiosk at our local mall. I also volunteer at a local shelter for the homeless and am involved in a wonderful church where we have close friends and fellowship. Some of my favorite things in life are; Bible study, the Green Bay Packers, classical music, jewelry, visiting art galleries, and craft fairs. I love taking road trips with my hubby, and all activities involving my grandkids.

I started graying when I was in my late teens, early 20's, and that's when I started coloring my beautiful black hair. It was gorgeous, and really, no one knew I had colored my hair, as it was very shiny and full of life. It was thick, naturally wavy, and the envy of many. I colored until my early

30's, when I finally realized that I had ruined every bathmat, towel, and tee-shirt in the house. Coloring my hair was a messy, smelly, and toxic process. I started to hate the tyranny of the whole scene. My colored hair no longer spoke of my reality, naturalness, and wholesomeness.

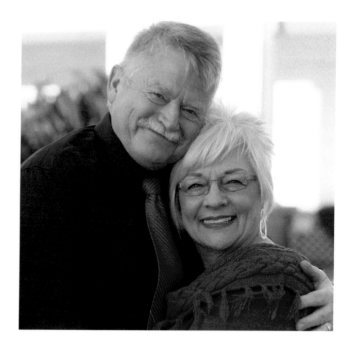

I just stopped coloring and let nature take its course—no angst, hesitations, fears, or hassles. My gray and white hair started out very slowly; then, by my mid-50's, things really got underway. That is when I found my face framed in gray, then silver, and now white. The back of my hair is still very salt and pepper.

I did have one crazy episode during this process, when I tried to hurry Mother Nature. I decided to have my hair stripped of all its color, thinking I would make it all white, but it turned out a horrible shade of yellow and looked like straw! What a mess that was! After that, my hair turned every color under the sun, and I had no recourse but to go for a cute pixie cut to rid myself of all that damaged hair. It gave me back my natural salt and pepper hair, and I discovered that I liked having short hair. Lesson learned: Do not mess with Mother Nature!

I cannot tell you how glad I am, to be a true silver sister. No muss, no fuss, and no more mess, just health, freedom, pizzazz, and a uniqueness all my own. I'm glad that I stopped coloring my hair early enough so that I didn't have a demarcation line, or a lot of people insisting that I color. I really love the ease of my natural color, and I have never regretted it for one moment. Happy transition! Hi, Ho, Silver!

GRAY8 TIPS & TECHNIQUES

I just love a product called TOPPIK! It's a white powder that I sprinkle on my pink scalp (right in front) where my hair parts and looks thinner. It really does make my hair look thicker, and gives it much more volume.

Brandee Bolden

Age 36
Ohio

I was in high school when I first started seeing those silver-gray hairs. Just like magic, they seemed to appear out of nowhere, but, at this point, a good pair of tweezers kept the grays at bay. As soon as one would appear, I pulled it out!

It wasn't long before I started coloring my hair for fun. My mom was a beautician, so I would end up being her guinea pig. I was able to try just about every color of hair dye imaginable! I enjoyed trying all the different colors, but my favorite was auburn. Then, one day, I decided to color my hair on my own. I dug out my box of auburn and proceeded. Well I'm not sure exactly what I did wrong, but my hair ended up looking like my scalp was bleeding! The dye grabbed my hair so strongly that, when I went to wash it out, I looked like the tip of a bright red crayon! That was the last time I dyed my hair red; from that point on, I decided to stick with a honey brown.

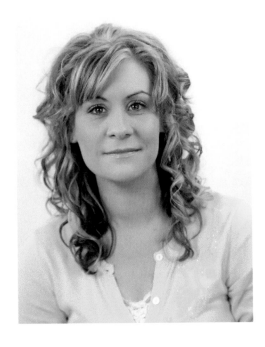

I stopped dyeing my hair towards the beginning of 2012. I had recently had my hair cut very short, as in, only a few inches long, SHORT! Having my hair this length, I soon realized how much gray I actually had. In just two short weeks, my silver streak would re-appear in my part. So I looked at this as the perfect opportunity to embrace the silver mane that the good Lord gave me to see where it would go!

Since I decided to cut my hair very short, it was easy to cut away at the dyed hair; and took only four short months to complete my transition. I was lucky that the crown of my hair was so white, because it looked like I had natural highlights. It took me two years to grow my hair to the length that I have now. I actually think it was harder for me to grow out my hair, than it was to go gray! Now I love my hair! I think that it is healthier and shinier than ever! The only thing I miss is changing my hair color on a whim. I have to tell myself, (as I walk through the hair color aisle at the store), that if I dye my hair, the only way to get the silver hair back, is to cut it off and start all over again. I don't want to do that!

After I let my hair go natural, I wondered what type of feedback I would get, but it has been overwhelmingly positive! I was really worried about what my eleven year old would think; I didn't want him to be embarrassed that his mom had hair like a grandma. But thankfully, he is one of my biggest supporters! When I joke with him that I'm thinking of dyeing it, he tells me no because he thinks it looks, beautiful!

try to keep my hair out of the sun by wearing a hat. The sun turns my hair yellowish!

As far as jewelry goes, I rarely wear gold, as I think silver is much more complementary with my hair.

I think dyeing my long brown hair blonde, and cutting my hair short, made the transition a little less noticeable.

Carol Ann Cheatham
Age 51
Michigan

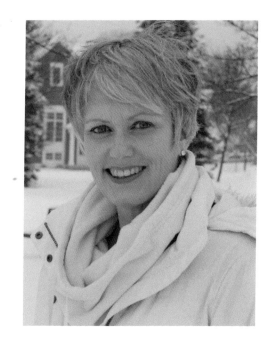

Well—I did it! After many months of discussion, consideration, and anxiety, I finally did it! IT... was... the decision to transition to gray. Almost everyone thought I was crazy. My husband did not want me to be gray. My fourteen year old daughter was appalled at the thought of her mother having gray hair. My friends questioned my sanity. And most people wondered why I would even consider giving up my highlighted medium blonde hair to be a gray-haired old lady!

I am a wife, mother, a business professional, and, all-around busy person. My hubby Rich and I have been married for almost 20 years. We have three children, ages (22), (17), and (14), and an Apricot Standard Poodle puppy. I play the flute in our local community band and love to do Bikram yoga. I am an avid reader and belong to a book club. Ironically, I am one of the youngest women in the club and the only one with gray hair!

I started coloring my hair at the age of sixteen. My first experience was with a product called "Sun In," which ended up turning my hair very orange. Then I talked my mom into letting me get highlights. This worked great for several years because I did not have to color my base. However, around my mid 30's, I had enough gray that it became necessary to color my base, too. Now I was doing highlights and a base color. I continued this process until, one day, I just decided I was done and went to all-over box color and became VERY blonde. Eventually, I went back to the base plus highlights because that gave me a more natural look. The whole hair color obsession was very time-consuming. I would pick through my hair and, as soon as I saw a few gray hairs, I would make my appointment for a touch-up.

It was exhausting, and expensive! Oh, and the damage! I hated the way my hair would fade to a brassy yellowish straw with silver temples.

My 50th birthday in 2012 would be the last time I did any base color. This was such a liberating decision. My hairdresser was on board and said that he would help me through the transition. He gave me a fun, funky shorter haircut, and I highlighted the brassy areas with white blonde to help blend it all together. I only had to highlight a couple of times. The frequent trims made the process go pretty fast. I was completely finished transitioning in eight months. I think that getting the highlights made the transition easier. Otherwise, I may have started coloring if the gray stripe was too dramatic.

A funny thing happened after I was done with the process. My hair stylist admitted that he was not so sure about my decision, but he loves the color now. My husband thinks it's sexy, and my mother is now considering her own gray transition. On a recent vacation to Savannah, strangers stopped me several times while walking down the street to discuss my hair. Crazy! I never got that much attention while coloring. The freedom that this decision has allowed me is difficult to describe. I just love having natural hair. For the first time in 34 years, my hair is healthy, and shiny, and it's all mine! It is silver instead of yellow straw. I feel pretty, sexy, and fresh, and I highly recommend going gray!

GRAY8 TIPS & TECHNIQUES

I use Aveda Blue Malva Shampoo and Conditioner. Once a week, I deep-condition with coconut oil and let it sit for fifteen minutes. I lightened my makeup, and made only a few minor changes in my wardrobe colors.

Cathy Graf
Age 55
Washington

I am a Washingtonian throughout. Born and raised in the Evergreen State. I have a great love of the outdoors, and grew up camping and backpacking. I met my husband Larry in my freshman year in Earth Science class. We met again in Chemistry class in our junior year of high school; we were Chemistry partners (no pun intended), and we've been together ever since. We have been married for 35 years and have two sons and a daughter. I also have three grandchildren, and love spending time with them.

My husband grew up boating, and I was introduced to boating at age seventeen. He bought a Hobie Cat, and we spent several summers racing Hobie's. Great fun! My other hobbies include; knitting, quilting, scrapbooking, bicycling, snowmobiling, snowshoeing, and walking. We have a cabin in the Okanogan Highlands at 4,000 feet, and, in the winter, I enjoy walking out the door to play in the snow. Sitting in a toasty cabin, sipping hot chocolate, and watching the snow fall, (is so peaceful), after playing all day in the snow. I also love animals. We have a sixteen year old Calico cat and an English Cocker Spaniel, who was my "empty nester" dog.

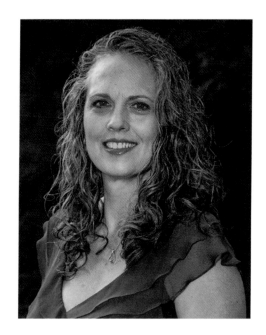

I was lucky to be a stay-at-home mom while working part-time for our business. My husband started his own boat manufacturing company 26 years ago. In 2007, he left the original company and started Aspen Power Catamarans. At this point in time, I perform a variety of tasks for our company. I created our website, design ads for magazines, do various clerical jobs, and sew the window coverings for our boats.

I started dyeing my hair about 1990. I had a handful of gray hair, and my stylist talked me into coloring. I did not like the contrast with my dark hair, so I started the cycle of dyeing. I was a profit center for her.

I was in the routine of going to a salon every six weeks for a cut, color, and foil. I spent around $150 for each visit, or approximately $1,200 per year. As time went on, I could not stand the grow-out. I thought it looked like tiny silver spider legs on the top of my head. In 2006, I was going to the salon every five weeks to cover up those spider legs. When I look back through my old pictures and see the colors my stylist was putting on my hair, I realize I looked hideous! I think the worst color was an orange and red concoction.

When we started our new boat company, I decided I just did not want to spend that kind of money on my hair anymore. I was tired of going to the salon every five weeks. So I had gray and silver highlights foiled into my hair and started the transition. I let it grow until the new growth was at the bottom of my ears and then had it cut into a bob. I have been growing it long ever since. Now I don't have fried over-processed hair that looks like hay anymore!

Sometimes I feel a little self-conscious that I don't dye my hair, especially if I'm in a group where I'm the only one that doesn't have dye on my hair. But I do get lots of compliments on my hair, too. My salt and pepper hair complements my skin tone, which my dyed hair didn't do. I'm glad that I'm not a slave to my hair stylist anymore. My husband loves my healthy, shiny, "salt and pepper" curly hair!

GRAY8 TIPS & TECHNIQUES

I'm a curly girl, so my hair is really coarse and dry, and frizzes easily. I co-wash; I get my hair wet and rinse conditioner through it. I have made my own conditioner, which works pretty well. No silicones or sulfates on my hair! I wash with shampoo about twice a week, and have used both DevaCurl and Jessicurl products. Once in a while, to prevent yellowing and remove any product build-up, I'll use a purple shampoo or baking soda wash with a white vinegar and water rinse. I let my hair air-dry. Using a blow-dryer seems to dry my hair out more and make it frizzy. I just discovered "hair plopping" online and find that I have more lift on top and that it enhances my curls to use this method after conditioning.

For clothing, I love wearing all the jewel-tones, which look great with gray hair! Right now, my favorite color is PURPLE!

To make my transition easier, I had my hair highlighted with gray and silver. Then, once my grow-out was past my ears, I had it cut short into a bob.

Debra Toutloff
Age 56
Canada

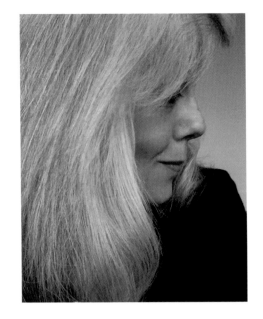

I was born in Toronto, the provincial capital of Ontario, Canada, and lived, studied, and worked there previous to the last five years. Now, home is living in a converted barn outside the city on a property that is almost 26 acres, growing wild. It is wonderful living in a giant meadow, seeing deer, wild turkeys, and birds of prey. It is so quiet I can hear myself think. It is so private I can take my morning coffee outside on a fine summer's morning, still in my PJ's, hair in its usual morning disaster, without fretting that anyone will see me, before I've gotten myself together for the day. What a change after living in a big city!

I am an artist—it's been a standing joke between my brothers and me since we became adults. They would often ask, "When are you going to get a real job?" You know—something you hate, but have to do, to pay the bills. I've been fortunate enough to have had the opportunity to do more interesting and varied things. I loved my stint in the world of advertising, working as a studio artist—at the agency I drew storyboards, which is what is used by creative teams to sell a client on television commercials. They are like drawing giant comic books. I've also free-lanced as an illustrator, and draw and paint for my own pleasure, as well. I'm old school—I love pencils, paint brushes, and canvas. It's the hand work that captivates me—the challenge of mastering the medium and teasing an image out from one's imagination.

I had a large break in terms of work when raising my three children. While I had stepped away, the industry I had known changed, not necessarily for the better. When I was ready to go back to work, quite by accident I discovered that my skills and imagination were an asset to doing fantasy and special effects makeup. My then-husband was a very conservative fellow and not in any way appreciative of my ability to create a character, or fashion a horrific wound with makeup. This really capped a lot of personal differences between us, and a long marriage came to a messy end. I loved the fun of the Halloween trade, a solid month of doing demonstrations and booking appointments for all the big parties and contests of the season. My current partner works as a Film Technician in the Electrics Department, so for his appointment (when we first met), I made him up to look like he had been electrocuted. He asked me out the very next day, and we have been together ever since—ten years now. Most currently, I am working on illustrations for a children's book.

I am not shy about painting myself, either! My hair has been many styles and colours over the years. Early on, it was just because I could; it was experimentation and fun. In my mid-40's, it became more about self-consciousness, the march of time and anxiety about projecting a certain image, since I was fearful of losing my footing in terms of employability. Once colouring became a have-to and a chore—it got old fast; it got to be work. I started seriously thinking that I would rather march to my own drummer and grow my grey hair out. It was a decision about freedom from what is expected, and the tyranny of deciding how to wear my hair, depending on where I was between appointments and how much of my roots were showing.

The last fifteen months, have been a time of transition—my true colour continues to shift and change, as the dye has been cut away and my natural mix of icing sugar, and chocolate, lengthens and softens. I still have moments when I look in the mirror and momentarily don't recognize the woman I see. I am still working on how to put together the new me. There is nothing better than coming to a place where you are at peace with the changes that maturity has brought you, when you stop fighting change and embrace it.

GRAY8 TIPS & TECHNIQUES

I wash my hair daily, and alternate between shampoo, and washing my hair with conditioner only. I use Pantene Pro-V Aqua Light Shampoo. Most often, I also add a very small amount of baking soda to my shampoo. Baking soda helps keep mineral deposits from building up on my hair, (since I have well water), and it keeps those silver hairs, light and luminous. Then, every ten days, I change my routine and use a violet shampoo and conditioner. After I rinse out my conditioner, I rinse my hair again with a diluted vinegar/water rinse, followed by one more quick rinse with regular water. This makes my hair very smooth and glossy. For frizz-free hair, I use Pantene Pro-V Smooth Serum with Argan Oil. It leaves my hair smooth and silky. I also deep-condition with extra-virgin coconut oil once every couple of weeks for about two hours. To dry my hair, I use a blow-dryer (set on medium heat), and often finish with it set on cool. During the warm summer months, I leave my hair a little damp and either French-braid my hair, or wear it up.

I found headbands and bandanas to be very helpful, during my transition. For me, cutting my hair short, made my transition go quickly.

Dede Watson Runnels

Age 48

Texas

I met my husband, Dr. Marti Runnels, online and have been married nine years. He is the Dean of Fine Arts at a university. I work full-time as a pharmacy buyer-technician at a local hospital, and also provide all the costuming for my hubby's theater programs. Between the two of us, we have three kids, one grandson, and a second on the way! We are 100 percent outdoorsy folks and enjoy hiking, climbing mountains, and kayaking! We look forward to our retirement years so we can live, travel, and work out of our RV.

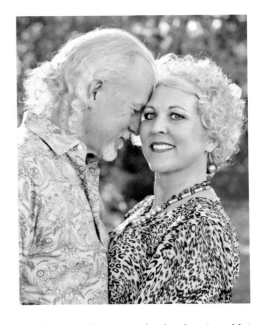

Like so many of us, I have been coloring my hair since I was in high school, trying to capture those platinum blonde streaks of summer with "Sun In." As a young adult, I started coloring my hair big-time. I would change it up according to the seasons, weather, mood, or amount of wine I had to drink!

Then the silver came in—and I was coloring my hair every three weeks. I was absolutely miserable! I would go to bed, and suddenly remember that I had a meeting the next morning, so I'd have to get up out of bed – a couple of hours early, just to color my roots!

Fast forward to age 43, when I had just began getting my hair colored at the salon again. The stylist had just applied the color, and I was sitting under the heat when it happened—my scalp was on fire, and I became nauseated! I could not get to my stylist fast enough—begging her to get the dye off my head! The results were horrifying. My entire scalp was a solid scab. According to my physician, I had developed a PPD allergy and would never be able to color my hair again!

So, with the help of my online friends and family, I began the transition process. My two sons were my only "nay-sayers," insisting that I would look older. My husband only questioned me once, before he got on my going gray bandwagon and, yes—he was already gray. Now, I get compliments almost daily on my hair! For the first time in my life, I feel like my hair color fits me, naturally and authentically!

GRAY8 TIPS & TECHNIQUES

For frizz and shine I apply virgin cold-pressed coconut oil on my hair, right after a shower. I also use Living Proof No Frizz Conditioner and Living Proof Nourishing Styling Cream.

For makeup I use Boom Cosmetics, then I just apply a little mascara and eyebrow color, and I'm done!

Denise Buchoz

Age 57

Texas

I am a print model living in the beautiful Texas Hill Country. I have been married for more than 24 years and have three adult children, a 34-year-old son, and 24-year-old twins (one boy, one girl). Both twins recently graduated college! I have also been gray for almost seven years!

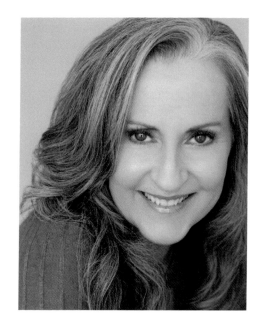

I first started noticing gray hairs on my head when I was around 21. It wasn't a shock for me because my mom and grandma were gray at a young age too. By the time I was 35, I dyed it because of the negative comments I received i.e., going gray would make me look old; I was too young to go gray etc. My natural hair color growing up was brunette, so that is the color I always dyed it. I got tired of dyeing it pretty fast, and stopped when I was in my 40's. I was curious to see what was under all that dye! Going gray was the best, most freeing thing—I have ever done for myself.

When I started the transition, I went to a salon to get my hair cut short. By the time I got home, the skunk line looked so bad that I decided I might as well just shave my head and start fresh. So I did. My advice to others who are considering going gray is: Be your own biggest fan. Be confident in yourself as your hair goes gray. I rocked a short, spiky look and a one-length bob as my hair grew out to where I wanted it. Another important transformation tip: You're doing this for yourself, not anyone else. Other's opinions or negativity can't be a part of your transformation.

Today, I am fully transitioned with incredible silvery hair, and it has been this way for almost seven years. I have healthy hair that goes all the way past my waist. In addition to being unique and owning my individuality through my hair, my passion is (and always will be) horses! I grew up showing horses, and my daughter started showing at age seven. I got lucky with that! I also have a working dog/model/actor named Lincoln. I am a very active person, I attend the local YMCA with friends five days a week doing yoga, kickboxing, and step class. I love the Austin music scene and love to "two-step" and dance all day! I enjoy hosting dinner parties at my home with friends and family, and making crafty things from Pinterest, as well.

I love being an inspiration to my daughter and her friends. Because of my going gray, they have grown up with a better perception of what going gray is all about. I'm still just as active and youthful, but a heck of a lot more distinguished and unique. I say, rock the gray!

GRAY8 TIPS & TECHNIQUES

I use Matrix Total Results So Silver Shampoo and Matrix Biolage Hydrating Shampoo. For my conditioner, I use Matrix Biolage Hydrasource. For leave-in conditioners, I use Matrix Total Results Miracle Treat 12 and TIGI Catwalk Curlesque Leave-in Conditioner for curly hair. I use no other products or sprays. I never use products like mousse, gels, or hairsprays. I have naturally wavy hair so I air-dry and leave it be for most of the time. I only use a blow-dryer or curling-iron when necessary for the haircut/style. I use a wide-toothed comb sometimes, but no brush. I also believe that if you take care of yourself inside, your hair and skin will show it. I also wear braids, ponytails, and fun vintage flowers and clips. I always get compliments; however I wear it, because of the unique color.

As far as makeup, before going gray I wore more browns and greens. After going gray, I started wearing much cooler colors like blues, pinks, purples, etc.

Denise O'Neill
Age 52
Northern Ireland

I didn't wake up one morning seven years ago and say to myself, "I fancy going grey today." Nor did I make a plan in my life that when I hit my mid-40s, I would stop dyeing my hair. No, it wasn't like that.

I had coloured my hair regularly since my mid-30s, with one of the well-known semi-permanent do-it-yourself hair dyes. You know, one of those products where you "imagine" that you could look just like the model on the box. And, although I never did look like the model, for quite a few years I did feel confident in the way it made me look. I didn't have very many grey hairs, just a few around my temples, but the dye hid them nicely, while giving my hair a lovely rich colour and texture. I felt that my hair looked good, until there came an "alarm bell moment," when I began to notice that I didn't look right, and some other factors came into focus too.

I was 45, and I began to notice that my dyed hair was becoming a harsh contrast against my face, which was emphasising my wrinkles and paler skin. It was actually sucking the life from my complexion, and making me look older. This was ironically the opposite of what I had been brainwashed into believing by the hair colouring ads. I observed too, that my hair was getting a little thinner, especially in front, and that my scalp was more visible through the dyed hair. (This is normal for women of the perimenopausal phase of life.) The frequency of the colouring applications was becoming frustrating, as I had to colour my hair every two weeks to hide the grey roots. I used to get three to four weeks duration from my hair colour—not any more. I resented putting chemicals onto my scalp, which might not be a healthy thing to do. So, I said to myself, "Stop fighting it; let the colour

beautiful, sassy, and confident. Usually, trends are set and promoted by the large fashion and beauty industries, and the consumer follows. But, my perception is that ordinary women are taking the lead in ditching the dye and becoming the trailblazers for grey.

I always say that if you go grey and you don't like it, you can always colour again. It really is that easy. You have nothing to lose and everything to gain. It's one of nature's best-kept secrets. I am looking forward to my ongoing journey and watching all the future changes to come with my natural hair colour. I don't know how my shades of grey are going to look as each year passes, but I love the fact that I don't know. It's going to be a lovely surprise—nature's gift to me! Grey hair should be perceived as just another colour, which is just exactly what it is! And—just a final word—because we are worth it too!

Photo credit: Gavin Byrne/Red River Studios

Donna Johnson
Age 53
Indiana

I work in the legal field for a large law firm, and I also coordinate several staff events. I have been in corporate work for about 21 years. I am the mother of two, a son and a daughter, and the grandmother of three young grandsons that I absolutely adore. I have been very blessed with a very loving and supportive husband and family!

I began dyeing my hair for fun when I was 21. By my mid-20's, I started seeing my grays come in more frequently. Then my dyeing for fun, turned into dyeing because I had too. Little did I know, the vicious cycle I was about to embark on, was nearly impossible to stop!

As time went on, I began to realize how much I disliked coloring my hair; it just became a chore. I hated the cost, the time involved, the smell, the upkeep, and the rashes that I would get around my neck after coloring.

As I approached my mid 40's, I was now getting my hair dyed every three weeks, and it was becoming nearly impossible to keep up with the roots, as they came in so quickly. Now I had to use hair mascara or something similar, just to keep up with my roots between appointments.

My curiosity about gray hair started over two years ago. My husband and I were out shopping at an antique/flea market, (something we have always enjoyed doing together). Suddenly, I found my husband talking to a woman who seemed to be in her early 50's. She had beautiful shoulder-length silver hair; it was absolutely gorgeous. My husband asked her if she would mind talking to me about her going gray experience. At first, I thought to myself, that although her hair was beautiful, there was no way that I could ever let my hair go gray. When she spoke to me, she was very matter-of-fact, but she said something that struck a chord with me: "It's only hair; if you don't like it, color it again." After that, it was as if a light bulb went off in my head. She was right. If I didn't like it, I could just color it, so when I went home that night, I started searching the Internet about going gray. I saw so many beautiful pictures of women with gray hair and enjoyed reading about their going gray journeys. It was not long after that I started my own going gray journey.

I stopped dyeing my hair on February 1, 2012, with the encouragement and support of my husband. I must admit it was not easy, especially since I choose to keep my hair long. But I love my hair now, and I have never looked back!

GRAY8 TIPS & TECHNIQUES

For hair care, I use DevaCurl Low Poo, One Condition, and Light Defining Gel. I've found these products keep my hair soft, less frizzy, and bring out my natural waves. I also use Joico Color Endure Violet Shampoo and Conditioner two-three times a month to tone down any brassiness. My best hair care advice is to condition and condition again; especially if you are choosing to keep your hair long, as the dyed part may start to turn brassy. I deep-condition my hair with coconut oil once every two weeks.

I suggest that you invest in headbands, hairclips, scarves, and anything else you can use to creatively help disguise your incoming roots, (not that the gray hair coming in is a bad thing), it is the contrast between the gray and the leftover dye that can make you feel self-conscious. You will find that at the different stages of growth, that some people find this difference "so cool," as several young women have told me. I also suppose some people were trying to figure out what I was doing with my hair and some thought I colored it that way on purpose.

I must admit that in all my years of changing hairstyles, the color of my hair, etc., I have never had so much attention regarding my hair, as when I started to grow out my natural color. The vast majority of the attention was positive. You will find in the earlier stages of going gray, that people seem to look at the top of your head, more than at your eyes, during a conversation. You may feel like your hair is the only thing that you ever think about, but I promise you, it gets better. You will get to a point where, unless someone mentions your hair, you don't even think about it. I never thought I would get to that point, but I did.

I avoided mirrors at all costs... just kidding (somewhat)! I just tried to focus on other areas of my looks, such as makeup, clothing, and accessories for my hair. I tried to, and still try, to stay current in fashion. I wear a little brighter lip color on most days; because I am fair, I think this helps me to personally feel better, maybe due to the contrast between my lighter hair color and the lip color. However, I am now starting to like warmer colors of makeup, as well.

Once you are gray, experiment with colors, and try not to limit yourself to what you "think" you should wear. If you feel good in what you are wearing in your makeup and clothing, then you will project that in your interactions with other people. There is no substitution (even hair color) for feeling good, treating yourself and others kindly, and projecting true happiness.

Dulcy Checkland-Huard
Age 61
Canada

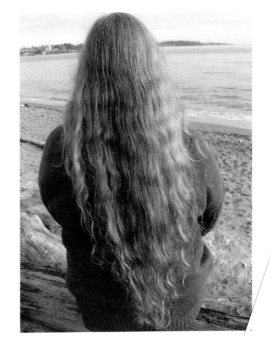

I wore a dyed short pixie cut for almost ten years, before I decided to go gray and let my hair grow long again. The dye no longer covered my temples, which had become colour resistant, and the salon would have to "pretreat" that area with chemicals—in order for the dye to take! My hair was brittle, brassy, and breaking off within a week after colouring it! My hair was also thinning rapidly!

To begin my transition, I first grew out my dyed layered hair to armpit length. I grew out my roots a few inches and did highlights twice over the next year to help blend things in. Then I just let it grow longer with no more colouring of any sort. It blended the dye demarcation line, and the highlights blended in well over time.

Minus a few trims to get rid of the layers, I never cut my hair short to transition. Instead, I grew it out longer and wore an Ombre look. In just four years, I went from a dyed orange-brassy short pixie, to almost tailbone-length, silver-streaked hair. Now I have white bangs, shoulder-length side layers that are also white, and a v-cut in the back to my tailbone, with lots of light brown and a silver streak in back. I love my hair! No more monthly salon cuts or twice a month dye jobs, and, as a bonus, my previously thinning hair has thickened up! I wish I had never dyed my hair and had done this much earlier than in my 50's! So much time and money were wasted, not to mention the years of using all those scary chemicals on my head.

I have very thick and heavy hair, so recently I went for the v-cut and am very happy I did! With this method, I still have my length that I had before, but without the heaviness. I did not do layers, but someone with much thicker hair could cut layers along with their v-cut. Now I can wear a ponytail again, and it won't pull and tug at my scalp.

I have been married for almost 40 years, and we have two adult children and a houseful of pets. We have a rescued feral cat, a ragdoll cat, two small Chihuahuas, and a Moluccan Cockatoo. I love to draw, do crafts, read, and do research on new health alternatives. To keep in shape, I enjoy walking, yoga, and weight training. I do all my own cooking from scratch, and I used to run a cake-decorating business from my home many years ago. We turned our front yard into a huge rock garden with drought-resistant plants, and our back yard into a huge veggie garden. We try to follow a simple life.

GRAY8 TIPS & TECHNIQUES

I use DevaCurl products for my curly hair and wash my hair daily using the "curly girl method." NO detergent, NO sulphates, and NO heat. I can air-dry my hair in fifteen minutes, by using a floor fan. I use a boar-bristle brush to smooth the hair surface to my shoulders only. Sometimes I use a shine serum. I have my hair trimmed once a year at a salon, but sometimes use a CreaClip between salon visits. I love hair accessories and use different exotic forks, spin pins, beak clips, flexi hair clips, and assorted African butterfly clips. I use a manual spider-shaped hair massager daily on my head to increase circulation, and I make sure to get 60 grams of lean protein in my diet each day. By doing all these things, my hair grows much faster and comes in thicker.

Helen Smith
Age 46
Scotland

I am the youngest of three children and grew up in a small town in Ayrshire on the beautiful west coast of Scotland. I've been married to Rob for sixteen years. We don't have children, though for many years we had pet rabbits, most of whom lived a life of luxury. After gaining my degree, I worked in Human Resources for a while before being diagnosed, (24 years ago), with CFS—Chronic Fatigue Syndrome, following Infectious Mononucleosis/Glandular Fever. Like many illnesses, (because nothing is visible), it's not immediately obvious to others that I am ill. I am very lucky to have a wonderfully supportive husband and family,

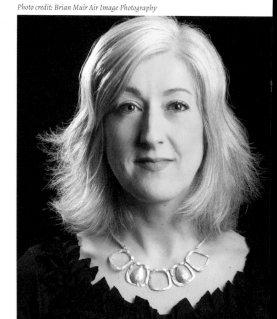

pioneers in this revolution; a new definition of what "true beauty" is, and the concept of aging and going gray. I am certain you will not regret your decision. Stay Sparkling Silver! Go Gorgeously Gray! Happy transition!

GRAY8 TIPS & TECHNIQUES

I use Jhirmack Distinctions Silver Plus Ageless Shampoo and Roux Fanci-Full (52) White Minx, (twice a week), to keep my hair from yellowing. My work as a model requires heat-styling-tools, and my hair is fine and scorches easily. A heat-protectant spray is a must. Also it's important to use a low-heat setting on your flatiron, curler, and dryer. I use a wide-toothed comb when my hair is wet, and a boar/nylon bristle brush works best for me when it is dry.

My advice is to be true to yourself, and not worry about the opinions of others. The support of a group like this is invaluable, and I only wish it had existed when I was turning gray! Break away from your norm, and experiment with new colors, new styles and new accessories; this is a time of change, and it's truly for the better!

Photo credit: Lynn Parks

Holly Barnett
Age 55
North Carolina

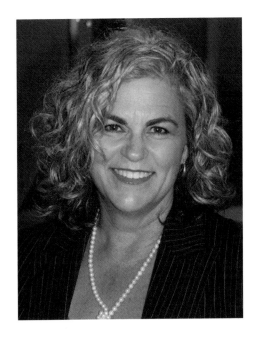

I grew up hearing the phrase "I love your hair!" Sometimes it was directed toward my own rich brown curls, but more often, it was directed toward my mother, who had a striking salt and pepper bob-styled cut. I still remember smiling, as one of my brother's friends referred to her as the "Silver Fox." People often stopped her in the supermarket to inquire about who did her color, or how her "frosted hair" looked so natural. Her answer? "It's all natural!"

So, with this background, one has to wonder why it took me five decades to take the plunge and go gray. My own silver streaks started in my 20's. I called them my credibility streaks, as I carved out a public relations career, where I sometimes felt a tad young, for the advice I was doling out. But as I entered my 30's, I caved in to the Southern California youth-forever culture, and regular trips to the colorist became part of my routine.

Eventually, that routine became an every-three-week ritual. Then, one day, my husband surmised that my mother's silver tresses might be hiding underneath all my artificial color. We had recently moved to North Carolina. I was working mostly from home and, frankly, knew very few people. "This could be the one time you could transition to gray, and no one will notice," he declared! So what the heck, I decided to give it a shot!

My stylist at the time was surprisingly supportive, and even pointed out that silver hair softens the appearance of facial lines that come with age, (or what I prefer to call wisdom, rather than age). We painted in some low lights to diffuse the skunk line, cut my hair into a cute bob, and started what would end up being an eight-month transformation.

I think my brother put it best when he said a year later, "I love your hair, but getting there was rough." So many times, I thought of giving up, but I'm so glad I stuck with it. Just about every day, I hear the same phrase my mother did when people stop me to compliment my hair color, and inquire about how I manage to have curly, frizz-free hair, on a humid North Carolina summer day, I smile and say, "It's all natural." If my mother was still here today, she would be very happy to know, that she paved the way.

GRAY8 TIPS & TECHNIQUES

I use DevaCurl products for curly and wavy hair. Recently, I discovered a local stylist (Scott Musgrave) who specializes in curly hair. He introduced me to water-soluble, silicone-free products that have helped me learn to embrace not only my natural color, but also my natural curl, another decision that I don't regret.

Janet Nuich
Age 58
Illinois

I was born and raised in Illinois. Growing up in the 60's and 70's, my first foray into the world of coloring was at the age thirteen, when I started using a product called "Sun-In." You sprayed it on your hair and went out into the sun to let it process. I liked the highlights it created in my medium brown hair, but in time they turned brassy, and I let them grow out. My next experiment in color came in my early 20's, when I decided I wanted to be a blonde, oh boy, what a bad experience that turned out to be! I went to a beauty school, where they stripped my hair, and, no matter what color toner they used, my hair still ended up platinum—and with my really dark eyebrows, I wasn't fooling anyone! By then, my hair was so damaged and dry that it actually started breaking off in chunks. Next, I went to a salon with a picture of my natural color, and, due to the extreme damage, it sucked up so much color that I went from almost white to black! Another bad experience, but eventually the color faded, and I went back and stayed with my natural hair color.

Then, in my mid-30's, I started seeing gray hair. At first, I would just pluck the strays out, but I soon realized that, like it or not, I needed them! Especially since I had fine thin hair, I needed every one I could keep a hold of. So I did what most women automatically do: I started coloring my hair.

As I aged, I would see more and more of the gray hair starting to show. I came very close to giving in a couple of times just to see what it would look like.

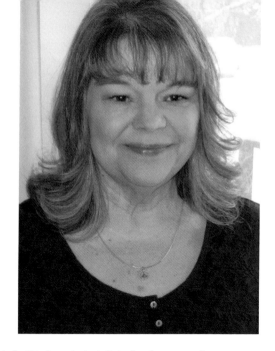

I would let about a quarter of an inch grow out and think, "No I can't do it!" And, of course, when I mentioned my thoughts to friends, they would respond with the usual, "It'll make you look old." "Gray hair is wiry." But I was still very curious! Then I found a book about "going gray" at the bookstore and brought it home. I admired all the women who were pictured in it, but decided I still wasn't ready to go there yet. So, I shelved the idea for a few more years. During those few years, I experimented with every hair color imaginable. One time, I even had a mixture of brown, blonde, and burgundy all at the same time!

Then my father was diagnosed with colon cancer, and I really starting thinking about all the chemicals we are exposed to every day, and it hit me like a lightning bolt! They tell pregnant women not to color their hair, and why? Because your body absorbs everything it is exposed to, and everything you put on it. When my father passed away, I decided to start my journey towards a healthier lifestyle, and going gray would be part of that journey. I was so ready to do this! I gathered up a few silver-haired pictures (of women that I admired) and took them with me to show my beautician. I wanted to speed up the transition process by dyeing my hair gray. Thankfully, she explained to me why that wouldn't work for me, but, more importantly, she did not try to talk me out of wanting to go gray. She helped me tone the color down so it would blend in better, and I had my last color in February of 2012.

After many trims and lots of support from my new Internet friends on several different sites, I cut off the last of the color in February of 2013 and have never looked back. I love the color, and the condition of my hair, and it has never been healthier or shinier. No more spending hundreds of dollars and hours trying to keep up with the never-ending cycle of coloring that begins the day after you color. I have adopted a healthier way of eating, as well, finally losing the many pounds I picked up along the way. Along with the transition, I have a new found confidence in myself and who I am and have made so many new friends along the way. I am having fun choosing clothing colors that complement my hair, and you know what? I found that all those tired old lines of "You'll look older with gray hair," etc., are just not true! I enjoy seeing all the transformations of my other silver sisters and brothers, and how vibrant and happy they all look. Mother Nature sure knows what she's doing!

GRAY8 TIPS & TECHNIQUES

To cleanse my hair, I alternate between Salon Grafix Healthy Hair Cleansing Conditioner and Paul Mitchell Tea Tree Shampoo and Conditioner. Once a month, I use Jhirmack Distinctions Silver Plus Ageless Shampoo and Conditioner, specifically designed for silver hair. Then, twice a month, I use one tablespoon of baking soda mixed in with my regular shampoo and rinse with a mixture of white vinegar and cold water to add shine. I also love Jhirmack Silver Brightening 5-in-1 Miracle Leave-In Treatment. When using a blow-dryer, I keep it on low heat, never going over medium. For extra volume, I blow-dry my hair with my head tilted down. Afterwards, I put a few Velcro rollers on top and leave them in while putting on my makeup.

I have made some wardrobe changes with my natural hair. I have found that I love colors that complement my hair, like navy, gray, silver, pink, dark red, and black. Wearing these colors lets me focus on more of a mix-and-match wardrobe, rather than the eclectic one I used to have.

Jeanne Marie Viviani
Age 43
Florida

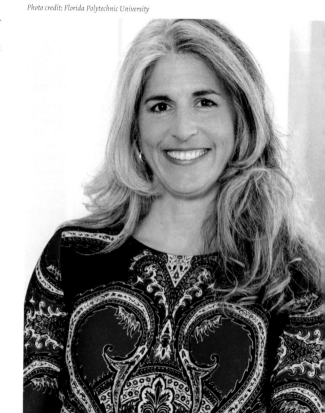
Photo credit: Florida Polytechnic University

Truth be told—I had my first gray hair at four years old! I come from a long line of silver and white hair, so being gray or silver or white was bound to happen sooner or later! My paternal grandmother was completely white by the time she was nineteen!

I started coloring my hair at age sixteen. I am the daughter of a hairdresser, so I always had access to the best hair products on the market. Since my hair grows like a weed, I was coloring it every two weeks, and of course, being Italian-American, I was coloring it dark brown.

Then in the summer of 2012, I decided I was done and went cold turkey. But at the same time, I promised myself that if I was going to go gray, that I had to make sure I wasn't going to have an "old body." So

I started back to weight training, too. It was funny how many people believed, after my hair was grown out about four inches (like in my competition picture) that I purposefully did my hair that way! I also did not want to cut my hair—I love my long hair.

I also had a lot of friends who questioned as to why I was letting my hair go natural. They thought it was a mistake, but now I get so many more compliments than I ever did, even from strangers! Friends are well-meaning, but trust your own image, and envision what you are inside and out! I'm lucky because I do have silver-white hair mixed with a few remnant strands of my dark brown (not the dye stuff).

I recently got married and have two beautiful daughters. I am the Contracts and Grants Manager at Florida Polytechnic University. I assist faculty with finding funding and managing their research portfolios. I also assist students with finding research projects to work on, and funding to do those research projects. I get to know students, and love my job! At a charity football game with the local college, my jersey said "Gandalf" on the back! Very fitting for advising and for my long gray hair!

I enjoy weight training, and, in June 2013, I competed in a Physique (like bodybuilding) competition. I had eleven percent body fat and was the "only" silver haired person out there! I also enjoy sitting on any one of the beautiful Florida beaches. I'm only about 20 minutes from Siesta Key, Anna Maria Island, and Lido Key!

GRAY8 TIPS & TECHNIQUES

I use WEN hair products. NO sulfates and NO harsh chemicals! They work great and leave my hair feeling silky-soft. I blow-dry my hair most of the time, but it also curls up nicely too.

Jennifer Seminara

Age 44

Arkansas

I am the mother of two teenagers, a daughter who is graduating high school and a son who is entering this fall. I grew up in the Midwest, and most of my roots are from rural Arkansas. Beans and cornbread is my thing! I went to college in New Jersey, where I met and married my husband. He came from a New York Italian-American family; so needless to say, I have come to love pasta! Twenty years later, our lives are crazy with jobs and kids. My husband became a Veterinarian, and I later became a Pediatric Cardiac Nurse. We moved to Arkansas to be closer to family. At my core, I am a science geek with a degree in plant biology. My kids grew up playing with my compound microscope and glass slides. In my free time, you will find me in my garden with grubby jeans and dirt under my nails. When I'm not covered in dirt, I paint or work on genealogy.

I vividly remember my first silver hair. I was 22 and living at a botanic garden in Pennsylvania. My

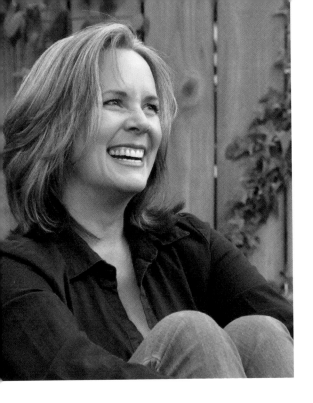

silver hair was about two inches long and, to me, absolutely beautiful. My roommate asked to see it, and, as I bent over to point it out, she grabbed it and plucked it out of my head. This was my first lesson in the fact that not all people appreciate silver hair!

I never had a negative opinion about silver hair. My dad's close friend, Meg, helped shape my perception of going gray. She is a free spirited, self-confident woman who to this day ranks among the most beautiful women I have ever known. She loves people and loves life. To her, going gray was something to celebrate; she was proud of who she was and was ok with the changes ahead. Meg had reached a point in life where she didn't want to color her hair anymore, and, in the few short years she and I were together, I watched her blissfully transition to silver hair. I remember her laughing, saying she couldn't wait to have a long gray braid. Life journeys moved us to different states, but when I saw her four years later, at my father's memorial service, she did in fact have the most spectacular long silver braid. I always intended to go silver naturally. In my mind, women with silver hair were like Meg; authentic, beautiful, proud, confident, and accepting of life changes.

In my early 30's, I noticed I was going gray a little ahead of my peers. A lovely stripe of silver was forming in my bangs. I had received a few off comments including, "Are you vitamin deficient?" So, in a weak moment, I decided to put a temporary hair color on to see how it would look. I failed to fully read the small print that said, "If this color is darker than your natural color, the results may be permanent." This began my ten years of coloring and highlights, because I wasn't sure how to stop. Sure, it looked nice, but it didn't feel like me.

In January 2013 at age 43, I made a commitment to stop coloring. I am the first of my peer group to decide to do this, and watching how others respond has been entertaining! I chose to start in the winter so my difficult period would be during the summer when ponytails were the norm. The first four months wearing a skunk stripe were the most trying for me. My hair stylist was extremely supportive and convinced me that the best course of action was to break up the transition line with some lowlights matching my base hair color, so I readily made an appointment. Unfortunately, in this one single appointment, she had covered up two months of my new growth progress! For the remainder of the year, I toughed it out and tucked, parted, and did whatever else I needed to do to survive my half-and-half look. I've just passed my one-year anniversary and still have brown tips, but the more silver my hair becomes, the more beautiful I feel.

My daughter, Emily, is eighteen years old, the age I was when I watched my dad's friend transition. I am excited to go silver, and happy that she is here to experience it with me. She has pondered what her own silver might look like someday and if she will turn gray early like I did. She said the other day, "I won't ever dye my hair. I mean, why should I?" That really made me smile.

It's comforting to see that my hair color is exactly like my dad's. I miss him and have made a commitment to take better care of myself and even added in a few hair vitamins. Now I am suddenly sprouting new hairs. I think the vitamins, along with not dyeing, have really helped my hair! My indoor hair seems to be mostly dark pewter with lighter streaks in a few places. In the sunlight, it is striking bright silver, and I love it!

GRAY8 TIPS & TECHNIQUES

I am naturally very oily and have very fine hair. My hair is easily weighted down and damaged by products. I use Pantene Pro-V Silver Expressions Shampoo; it has a purple tint to it. I condition every time I wash my hair. Regardless of what products I use, I make sure they don't have a yellow tint to them. For a great hair care treatment, I use Kevin Murphy Young Again Immortelle Treatment Oil. Unlike many silver heads, my hair does not like coconut oil at all! It felt stripped and damaged afterwards. I do, however, keep white vinegar in my bathroom, and, about once a week (if I remember), I do a vinegar rinse. My dilution is ten-parts-water to one-part-vinegar. It's an easy regimen, and, so far, my hair has looked healthy, soft, and shiny.

During the first few months of my transition, my naturally wavy/curly hair, proved to be most flattering in blurring the demarcation line.

Jenny Johnson
Age: 44
Minnesota

I was born and raised in northern Minnesota, and the youngest of three girls. After high school, I went even further north and attended Bemidji State University. After getting my social education for two years, I decided I needed to get serious and figure out what I was going to do with my life. So I moved to the Twin Cities at the ripe old age of 20 and started X-ray Technology School.

I always wore my hair natural until I turned 23; that's when I decided I wanted to have the Mrs. Robinson look from the movie, "The Graduate," dark shoulder-length hair with blonde streaks around my forehead and along the sides of my face. That was one of the longest hair appointments I've had to date. I loved my hair this way and got a lot of compliments on it. A couple years later, I decided to go from the sun-streaked mousy brown hair to jet-black. WOW! Talk about a dramatic change. As the

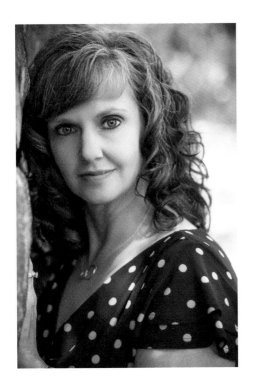

black was growing out, I began noticing the dreaded grays, at age 25.

For years, I wore my hair in every style and color imaginable, from bleached blonde and super-short to high-lighted and super-long past my shoulders. If I could add up the amount of money I spent getting my hair done, it would probably be enough to put my kids through college! Coloring my hair had become an every eight week ordeal.

It was in January 2013 that I finally decided I had been chemically dependent long enough. At this juncture, I was having my hair colored a dark brown shade, with occasional caramel highlights put in. I began talking to my stylist and told her that I was contemplating letting my hair go natural. She was very excited for me, and, together, we plotted what course of action to take. She suggested using very few demi-permanent color highlights to get me started.

As I started to see the gray coming in more prominently, I freaked out! OMG, I have to call and get my roots fixed! I was still going to the salon every eight weeks for trims and a color consultation/pep talk. My stylist was very supportive, and I couldn't have gotten to this point without her! The last time she touched-up my hair was in October, and, since then, it's been growing out very evenly; luckily, my hair grows like wildfire! That first time I walked out of the salon with only a haircut and an extra $50 in my pocket was a very strange feeling, but a very liberating one!

In early December, my husband and I were in Minneapolis for my employers Christmas party. We had lunch at a very popular hole-in-the-wall burger restaurant. Our waitress was probably about ten years younger than me, and, when she came to take our order, she said, "I love your hair, what do you do to it?" Not knowing if she was referring to the fact that I was wearing my hair stick-straight as opposed to my natural waves, I said that I used a flatiron on it. She said, "No, the color; do you have it colored, or is that your natural hair color?" I told her that it was all me, and she replied very enthusiastically, "I love it—it's just beautiful!" I thanked her and immediately sent a text to my stylist, telling her about the compliment. It really helped cement my decision to grow out my hair.

I have been living back in my hometown for about fourteen years, and I work as a medical receptionist for a very prestigious medical practice in Duluth, Minnesota. I've been married for eleven years and am the mother of eight year old boy/girl twins. Sometimes I think that I may get mistaken for their grandmother as opposed to their mother due to my hair being gray, but I'm really happy with how my hair is growing out. I have a lot of support from friends and family, especially my husband and my mother, who has seen every single hairstyle I've ever had!

Go forth with confidence, and be who you are and say what you feel. Because those who mind don't matter and those who matter don't mind!

GRAY8 TIPS & TECHNIQUES

I wash my hair twice a week and use Fructis Pure Clean Shampoo and Conditioner. As of yet, I don't use hair products specifically designed for gray hair, but will when the time comes. My hair is so thick that it takes hours for it to completely air-dry, but I prefer not to use a blow-dryer. For styling I use either a flatiron or big-barrel curling iron.

I still have some brown left in my hair, so I haven't changed my makeup at all. For clothing, I stick with solid colors; black, brown, red, and white are my favorites.

The best advice I would give to anyone considering this journey, would be to make sure that you have a stylist who will support you 110 percent! It makes all the difference in the world! Don't let public opinion dictate what you feel like doing to your hair.

Photo credit: Stephanie Beadle

Jo-Anne Neilson
Age 56
North Carolina

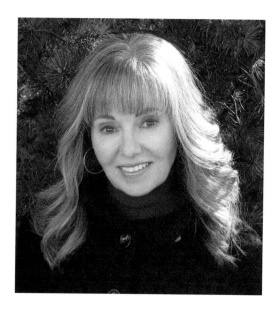

Unlike many women, I was someone who aspired to be a silver sister at a relatively early age. Nothing would turn my head more than a glorious mane of beautifully-styled gray hair. In college, one of my young classmates was completely and unapologetically gray, and I knew right then, that that was something I wanted for myself. It didn't hurt that she was model-pretty and one of the best dressers at school! My desire to go "au naturel" never wavered; it was just a matter of "when."

I've never had the hang-up of equating the color of one's hair to age, so that was not a hurdle for me. As my 50th birthday approached, and

I had become extremely allergic to the PBD's found in all hair dye, I finally felt I had enough gray to go for it. I was beyond excited to start this journey. Having dark auburn hair and not wanting the dreaded demarcation line, I chose to get a full head of platinum highlights. The first three months were easy; I even enjoyed my stint as a blonde, but certainly not enough to maintain it. Then, as the gray roots really started to show, I have to admit I didn't always feel that I looked my best. I had a wedding to attend, and I agonized over what to do with my hair. In the end, I decided to wear a fedora, and I received nothing but positive comments. Problem solved. Hats were the way to go for dressy occasions.

All in all, it took roughly eighteen months to complete the transition, and I'm never, ever, going back to dyed hair. I am a transplanted Canadian living in the US South, and women in this part of the country hang onto their colored hair like grim death. Occasionally, one will compliment me, but then quickly add that she could never do it herself. When I press for a reason, it's either, "My gray hair would probably not grow in as nice as yours," or "My husband wouldn't like it." As far as growing in nicely how do you know if you don't try? My experience has been that men absolutely love gray hair. By far, the most compliments I've received have come from men; especially young ones. Several men have told me they wished their significant others would stop dyeing their hair and therefore stop revolving their lives around salon visits. Can I get an Amen?

Update: I am three-and-a-half years dye-free now and basically retired, although I occasionally help my husband with his business. My passions are painting, mixed media art, and any form of dancing. I intend to start back with ballet classes after the New Year.

If asked what my three biggest accomplishments have been over the past two years, I would say:

1. Writing and delivering the eulogy at my father's funeral.
2. Experimenting with my art in a more fearless way.
3. Getting my driver's license at age 55!

GRAY8 TIPS & TECHNIQUES

My favorite hair products include Dove Oxygen Moisture Shampoo, Pantene Pro-V Beautiful Lengths Strengthening Conditioner, and Tresemme Tres Two Hairspray.

If you are currently transitioning to gray, and don't want to go the highlight route, may I humbly offer you a piece of advice? As much as you may think everyone is scrutinizing your roots, believe me, they are not nearly as fixated on them as you are! Repeat the mantra, this too shall pass, and keep your eye on the prize; glorious, authentic hair, just the way nature intended.

Julie Fisk

Age 56

New York

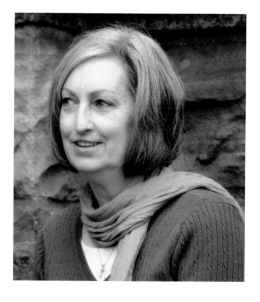

I was always a brunette, but as the "battle of the roots" became more of an issue, I decided to go blonde with highlights. For the next couple of years, I touched-up my roots at home, but went to the salon twice a year for the highlights. My journey into silverhood began right after my last salon visit in the spring of 2012. I was due to renew my driver's license, and since a new picture would be taken, I wanted to be sure I looked good. Especially since I would have this picture ID for the next ten years! How I wish now, that I didn't have a blonde stranger's face on that license!

I considered going gray for a few years, but when I started needing color every three weeks, I knew it was decision time. Do I keep on going and run to the store for more hair color? Or do I let myself go gray? The more I began to put the idea out there to family and friends, the more I heard all the gray hair clichés. "You are too young!" "It will make you look old!" "You won't like it!" But deep inside, I kept having the urge to find out what my non-dyed hair would look like. What if it looked really cool and I was missing out on it? Besides, if I didn't like it, I could always just color it again.

I finally made up my mind and decided to give it a try. It was scary and exciting at the same time. As the gray roots began to show, I felt as if everyone must be staring at them! I began constantly checking myself out in the mirror to see how I was progressing. I found a support group online, where I met other women who also wanted to go gray. We supported each other's journey and shared helpful hints that we found worked for us.

I work in an office for my local town government, so I am in contact with the public on a daily basis. At the time I started going gray, there were six other women working in our small town hall. They all began to watch me with interest. I even had one co-worker friend who decided to take the gray journey along with me! Our hair was very similar in coloring, so we had fun guessing what we would end up looking like.

In the beginning of my transition, I kept the same hairstyle, which was a stacked bob. In December, I was sporting two and a half, to three inches of skunk stripe. So much of my new gray growth was hidden beneath the long top layers. I was getting excited to see more of it. The blonde had long since turned brassy and looked awful against the shiny tones of silver and gray. For a few months, I found that using a product called Roux Fanci-Full Rinse in True Steel helped a lot. It is a rinse that will tone your hair color, but washes out with shampoo. It helped tone the brassy yellow blonde ends, into more of an ash-blonde. This blended much better with the gray strands.

Then, one day, I got the notion that I was tired of waiting to be done. So I took the scissors out and gave myself a haircut, putting layers throughout. I was so excited to see the dyed blonde hair fall to the floor. When I finished cutting, I was left with only blonde on the last half-inch of my hair and mostly on the crown portion. Everyone loved the cut and couldn't believe I had dared to do it myself!

On January 25, 2012, I went in for a salon graduation cut. In retrospect, had I realized how much my stylist would need to cut off for me to complete my journey, I would have waited a while longer. I left the salon that day with a mixture of emotions. I was happy that I was fully transitioned and all naturally gray. But I was very unhappy with my cut! I actually cried on the way back home because it was shorter than I ever dreamed of being, or was comfortable with.

This year has been one of growing the length back out. I have had such positive responses to my natural gray hair. My friend and co-worker completed her transition about two months after I did. During my transition I was unaware that others were watching me as well. I am happy to say that one woman from my church, and another from my extended family, have both made the transition. They told me that I was their inspiration, and that I gave them the courage that they needed to go through with it. Now, I have another friend three months in, and another church member thinking about taking the plunge. It feels fabulous to be all natural and an inspiration to others! I love my gray hair and am so glad I made this journey!

GRAY8 TIPS & TECHNIQUES

For toning and blending (during my transition), I used Roux Fanci-Full Temporary Color Rinse: White Minx (52). Another favorite product is Matrix Total Results So Silver Shampoo. Consistent hair trims and shaping will give you a cute style during your transition. Remember, people may be looking at your roots—but not for the reason you think. You too, might be just the "inspiration" they are looking for!

Kama Frankling
Age 46
Sunshine Coast, Australia

In 2011, I was not feeling my best. I suffered from numerous food allergies, headaches, aching muscles, and fatigue, and I had put on five kilos that just wouldn't budge. A visit to the doctor also revealed that my liver was failing, and something needed to be done quickly. To cheer myself up after seeing the doctor, I went to get my hair coloured. While sitting with the dye on my head, I began to feel a burning sensation, more so than I usually did. After fifteen minutes, I was desperate for the hairdresser to rinse off the hair dye. Although reluctant at first because the hair dye had not yet taken properly, the hairdresser finally paid attention, and rinsed off the dye. I left the hairdresser with a burning and stinging scalp that resulted in sores, and a swollen, puffy face. I had dyed my hair for more than 20 years, and I had always felt that there was a slight stinging sensation, but now this? Was I making a fuss, or was hair dye dangerous? So I started researching. My research showed that several of my health symptoms could be related to my reaction to the hair dye.

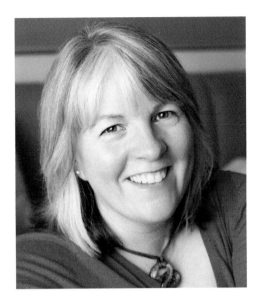

So, with much initial resistance, I decided to stop colouring my hair. Within just a few months two remarkable things happened:

1. All my health issues went away! Yes, all of them! Within five weeks, my liver was back to normal, my weight dropped, and I could eat whatever I liked. The doctor was more than surprised at my health improvements. I am still healthy.

2. I noticed that allowing my hair to be its natural colour was a journey to my own true inner confidence. Although I had thought of myself as reasonably confident for years, I also realised I had used my hair as my excuse to hide. I thought that as long as my hair was coloured and cut nicely, then all would be well, and I would feel reasonably attractive. If only I had known earlier how wrong I was! On my journey to silver, I discovered an inner confidence that I never even knew existed. I now love my hair. I love that the shades of silver/white/grey are forever changing. I love that I can now be who I truly am. No more hiding, no more pretending.

Now, as I look back on my experience, I wonder how many women are suffering from allergies and other health issues that could be related to hair dye. I am convinced that the numbers are much higher than we are aware of. What I find just as disturbing, is the number of women who are aware of the health issues related to them dyeing their hair, yet still feel pressured to continue colouring. I have also met so many women who are so health-conscious that they eat organic foods, use natural cleaning products, make their own beauty products, and yet still dye their hair with chemicals.

There is so much pressure to dye our hair. I wonder, though, where does the pressure come from? We say the pressure to dye is from society, yet we "are" society. So, in reality, we are putting this pressure on ourselves. What if we stopped believing that grey equals old, unlovable, and unemployable? What if we all stopped pretending that we have to be anyone other than who we truly are?

I am so happy to now have my health back and the freedom to be just me. I would love for many more women to know that freedom. I promise your life will not become dull and boring if you stop colouring; in fact, you may find your life improving as you reconnect with your true inner self. This journey is so much more than a change in hair colour. I can honestly say that no longer dyeing my hair has changed my life for the better.

I was born in the UK, but I call Australia my home. I have spent the past 30 years of my life living in various countries. I have lived in East Africa, New Zealand, Canada, Norway, The Netherlands, and Singapore. All my travels led to my first book, "The Happy Migrant," a step-by-step relocation guide for coping with the emotional aspects of moving.

Writing my first book gave me the writing bug. So I took notes of my experiences, my worries, and my growing confidence levels on my journey to grey hair. I felt that my notes, along with my experience as a counsellor and coach, could benefit others who wish to take this journey and yet don't quite dare to. This led me to write "Daring to Be Grey," how to confidently stop colouring your hair. I have been on what seems to be a long journey to find simplicity in my life, and now I am living an almost stress-free life. Check-out my new book "Stop Stressing Start Playing." You can follow my blog at http://www.almoststressfree.com.

When I'm not writing, I love to take photos of nature. I have a passion for nature and creativity, and I love to combine the two in my confidence sessions with clients. In my spare time, you will find me taking photos of flowers, walking in nature, painting, or jotting down my creative ideas. I don't like to take life too seriously, so you may also find me outside blowing soap bubbles or being a bit silly.

GRAY8 TIPS & TECHNIQUES

I use as many natural hair products as possible, and use very small amounts. If my hair yellows a little, (which often depends on the water used), I will add a very small amount of baking soda to my shampoo. If my hair is feeling dry, I apply a small amount of leave-in conditioner or Argan Oil. I deep-condition with coconut oil once a month and stay away from heat-styling tools.

A great hair tip is to eat nutritional foods. Just as your confidence comes from the inside, so does your health and well-being. If you are eating healthy whole foods, I guarantee you that your natural hair will shine. People said to me that my hair would no longer be soft and silky if I went grey, but this really isn't true! In fact my hair is healthier, bouncier, and silkier than ever before. I am obviously very health-conscious after my hair dye health issues.

Kate Leser

Age 53

North Carolina

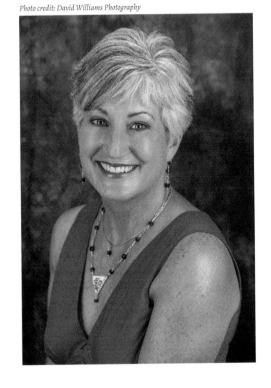

My first gray hair appeared out of nowhere at the age of 21, but I did not start coloring until my early 30's. I continued coloring until seven years ago. Going gray was not just about being free of the hassles of hair coloring, but more about honoring my beloved mom. I was always told that I looked like my mom, so when I lost her to breast cancer, I figured the best way to honor her memory was to let the gray shine through. You see, my mom was one of those powerhouse women who lived life to its fullest without worrying about what others thought of her. She was not only courageous, but kind, super generous, and totally natural. She was just being her. Now I am just being me.

I love my gray hair! I can hardly remember what it was like to have brown hair. The maintenance is minimal. I find that the gray is such a positive attention-getter! Compliments about my hair come from people of all ages, all races, and both genders. Grocery stores, football games, shopping malls, walking down the street—you name it, I get kudos all the time! After seven years, I still giggle at the attention, but I am much more accepting of it.

Just be you. What does that mean? To me, just being me is not using chemicals or dyes in my hair to create an illusion that I'm younger than I am. I am me; 53-years-old and loving myself as a gray-haired woman. Obviously, others love it, too, because I am still receiving, compliments, almost daily. As a matter of fact, last night, I received an unsolicited compliment from a young lady! My gray hair is who I am, so that naturally brings out the best in me, of which others are very accepting.

Going gray was one of the best decisions that I have ever made. I have more time for things I enjoy, I have little-to-no hair maintenance, and I am chemical-free. Most of all, going gray has been a liberating experience that allows me to be true to myself. I stand out in the crowd in a positive way, and I feel great about being me. What are "you" waiting for?

GRAY8 TIPS & TECHNIQUES

Are you worried that people will think you're older than you are? I'm not! There are three secrets to staying youthful and natural with your gray locks:

1. Take time to care for your skin in order to keep it supple and youthful.
2. Get a haircut that flatters your face shape, as well as complements your hair's texture.
3. Wear colors near your face that brighten your skin tone but that don't overwhelm your new found "lightness."

My favorite hair product is Catwalk True Wax by TIGI; it adds shine and keeps my hair in place.

Kate Mantz
Age 36
Wisconsin

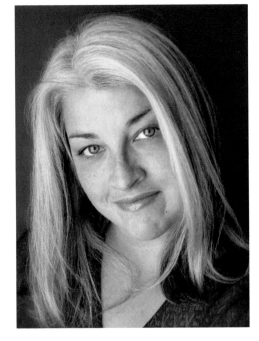

I remember I was only fifteen, when I looked in the mirror and saw my first gray hair! But, it wasn't until my early 20's that I started putting color on it. I never went through that dyeing for fun stage. When I started coloring, it was totally out of need. I continued to dye my hair dark brown until I reached the age of 30, and then, in November 2008, I decided that was it! I'd had enough, so I decided to STOP DYEING and START LIVING.

I decided to go gray mainly because I grew tired of the upkeep, the time that coloring involved, and the effect it was having on my pocketbook. I needed to get my hair colored every three to four weeks, just to keep up with my roots. The smell was terrible, and the staining of my scalp was torturous, rather than pampering.

I started out by having light blonde highlights put in my dark brown hair. From there, I just let it grow from November to March. To get me through my transition, I wore hats, headbands, and ponytails. Mix that in with a lot of determination and patience, and I was well on my way to destination gray! Then, on March 15, 2008, I cut my hair to a gray short pixie. It was awesome!

I love the length of my hair now. Having it past my shoulders, I am able to do a lot with it. I love the different ways I can wear it up, but I also enjoy wearing it down too. I get compliments nearly every day on my gray hair—much more so than when I was dyeing my hair. I feel very unique! It is not every day that you see someone in their 30's, with gray hair. I feel very fortunate that I was able to make this decision early on in my life, and was able to appreciate my true authentic self. Going natural was so liberating. My advice for anyone wanting to go gray is to be confident in who you are and go for it!

I have been married for eleven wonderful years and am a busy full-time mom to four kids, ages ranging from three to thirteen. I also work part-time as an Occupational Therapist. On my days off, I love to cook and bake, garden, and enjoy working on home improvement projects with my husband. I also enjoy spending time with the family and love all things gymnastics!

GRAY8 TIPS & TECHNIQUES

My hair routine is very simple; I use Suave Shampoo and Conditioner, and wash and condition my hair every other day. Rarely do I ever blow-dry my hair, and if I do, it is on a low heat setting. To finish up, I use a shine serum on my ends.

Kay Jones Brooks
Age 64
Alabama

My mother and dad both grayed early on in life, so I am confident that my genes dictated my future hair color or lack thereof.

A comb-over (not to be confused with an attempt at hiding loss of hair), was the method I used to try and hide my gray streak. It was an inch wide, and located just to the left of my center part. I was told time and again, that I must have a vitamin deficiency, or that I was possibly hit on my head (in that spot), to cause such a problem! This was 1967 during my senior year of high school.

In my early 20's, I decided to put a rinse on my hair to cover that gray streak. It would be a do-it-yourself dye job, something I knew very little about. And my gray streak turned orange! At a beautician's suggestion, I let her frost my hair to cover the orange, but after only one time, I decided to let it grow back out. It was a painful process!

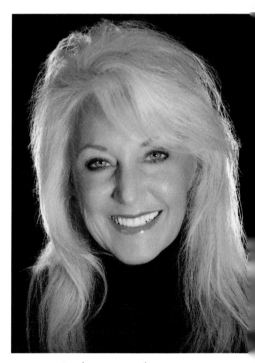

At 26, I had my only child, and that was when my hair really started graying all over. I wasn't crazy about the color back then; it was white in front, with salt and pepper everywhere else. The texture of my hair was changing also, and I found it difficult to manage, which was unlike my not so-long-ago straight, fine hair. Now it was wavy and unmanageable.

Around my mid-to-late 30's, I had a weak moment, and wanted to dye my hair. After considerable conversations with my long-time stylist who loved my silvers, I finally talked him into it. The Friday before my Saturday appointment, my stylist passed away—very early in life, and totally unexpectedly. I was saddened and still miss him to this day. I took Mike's death as an omen, not to go the dye route, (which he never wanted me to do anyway), and I decided to embrace my silvers!

Back when I decided to go gray, there were no social media sites on which to acquire information, or talk to others who were dealing with the same issues. I would walk up and down the aisles at drug stores, looking for solutions to my new problems of frizz, uncontrollable curls, and yellowing. I muddled through those years, (thinking I was all alone with these problems), buying every product I could find, (but not for gray hair), because you just couldn't find products for gray hair back then.

The years passed by with more and more white showing up, and the brown color, I had across the nape of my neck, was getting darker and darker until it looked almost black. I had to redefine my makeup so that I didn't look washed-out. In the beginning, I started by using a strategically placed self-tanner on my face for color and definition, and added additional color to define my eyes. I changed the colors of clothing I wore to deeper tones. I omitted brown, which I always loved, but no longer looked good in. It was an evolution, and I really started enjoying the challenge.

I love my hair, even though I still deal with the frizz, curl, and yellowing. The difference is that now I can use the Internet for research and find informative social media groups that I wish had been there during my formative years. I would suggest joining a gray support group for ideas and helpful information.

As a silver sister, I am very fortunate, and have never had anyone make a negative comment about my hair or my decision to go gray. Instead, I get compliments all the time; from family, friends, and even strangers who tell me how much they love my hair! I took great strides in my overall appearance and keep my makeup and clothing current. Everyone has always been so positive and supportive. Maybe this is because as my hair changed, I changed! I did not let my gray hair define me as old, not for one minute! Life is good!

GRAY8 TIPS & TECHNIQUES

I use Jhirmack products for silver hair, and my favorite product is Jhirmack Silver Brightening 5-in-1 Miracle Leave-In Treatment. In the White Hot Hair line, I use Shooshing Cream and Lifeshine Oil. I use Argan Oil for additional shine. One of my favorite go-to products is TOPPIK (a fiber used to cover areas of the scalp). I use the white fibers and love how they cover my pink scalp, through my transparent white hair.

Kaylee Nuttall

Age 39

Chester, UK

I have lived all my life in the city of Chester, well-known for one of the best preserved "Walled Cities." It is rich in history with its Roman Amphitheatre, Medieval Buildings, Gothic Cathedral, Chester Rows, and the Roodee Racecourse, (still in use today), and, according to official records, dates back to the sixteenth century. It is, without a doubt, one of the most attractive racing venues in the world.

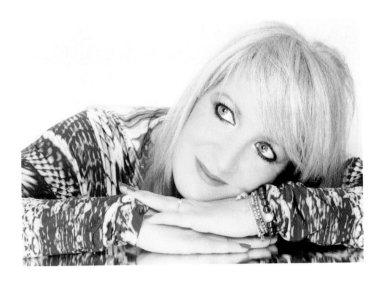

My partner and I have three wonderful children: a daughter and two sons. Our family also includes two Siberian Huskies. I work in retail in a well-known clothing shop and love spending time with my family and dogs. One of my favorite things to do is watch my son play football. (He recently became a scholar at Manchester City FC.)

My silver journey began back in 1985 at the tender age of eleven years old. To be honest, it has never bothered me going silver/grey early. One of my aunties (my mum's sister), who lives in Canada, was also silver at a very young age. So, seeing the few odd silvers peeking through on my natural dark hair came at no great surprise. Sometimes I would sit and pull at the odd one, and my friends and family would say, "Don't pull them out, or you will grow three more" (an old wives tale). Oh, boy, and how they were right! Look at me now!

Like most young women, I started messing around with hair colour in my teens. I first started out by using henna's at home. Using a wash-in, wash-out method, this would make my silver streaks a bit lighter in tone. I also experimented with other colours, depending on what colour hair I wanted to be that week! Soon I progressed to permanent hair dyes. Then, one day, I decided I wanted to be blonde. I bleached my hair, and it turned out a corn-yellow with orangey tones. It was a disaster! I quickly sent my older sister out to buy a box of dark hair dye. She applied it to my hair while laughing at me the whole time. What had I done? That's when I decided, "No more hair dye!" I did find it quite easy to grow out my silver hair, as it came through like streaks, and because it's quite long, I would just tie it back into a pony tail or wear head bands That was five years ago, and it has been one of the best decisions I have ever made for myself. Why not just stand out from the crowd and be unique? Let your silver hair shine! Don't GIVE UP or GIVE IN to the dye. Be confident, and be proud of who you are! It will be worth it in the end!

GRAY8 TIPS & TECHNIQUES
To remove any yellowing and to brighten my hair, I use Pro:Voke Touch of Silver Brightening Shampoo and Conditioner. On my ends I used Schwarzkopf Live Color XXL Ultra Brights 95 Electric Blue, and 93 Shocking Pink Semi-Permanent Hair Dye.

Kitty Kuzak
Age 65
Ohio

2009 was a year of change for me. I turned 60, I married for the second time, and I stopped coloring my hair. I accepted turning 60, with not a lot of fuss. Getting married was fantastic. BUT, to stop coloring my hair, well—that was downright scary! I had long blonde hair, and decided to go cold turkey. I threw my stash of hair color in the trash, and I let the journey begin. As the silver slid down my head, it was amazing to see all the colors that nature had given me. At ten months, I had my hair chopped to just above the collar. I remember how I felt the first time I saw the back of my head totally gray. My thoughts ranged from, "Yeah I did it!" to "Feeling a bit old, and missing my youthful blonde hair."

The transition was hard, although I have never been tempted to return to coloring. My goal was to have long silver hair, so I was totally looking forward to seeing what color I would actually be. Now, at four years being dye-free, I have to admit the scary decision to stop coloring my hair was one of the best decisions of my life. Although long silver hair comes with a certain amount of controversy, this is what I want and who I am.

"Live imperfectly with great delight." That simple sentence changed the way I lived my life. It seemed to be giving me permission to allow myself the freedom to be me and to stop trying to be perfect to please others. I was 60 at the time, and the last five years have been the most freeing of my entire life. This attitude also plays into my love of gardening. I have a garden full of flowers that look like the seeds fell from heaven, completely imperfect and utterly delightful.

My husband and I have enjoyed traveling this

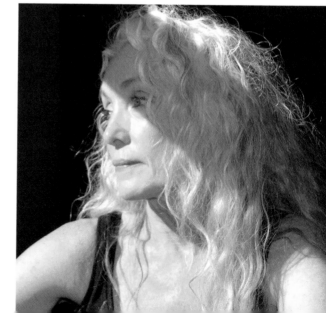

past year and spent four months in England. This has been a life-long dream of mine, and he made it come true. We met my senior year of high school, and, although we never dated, we never forgot each other. I moved away right after graduation, married, and had one child. My ex-husband and I eventually divorced, and, about a year later, I received an email regarding my high school class reunion. We met again, and slowly built a great friendship, which turned into a deep love for each other. My husband's encouragement and support, along with my own strong desire, got me to where I am today. I wear my white hair long, to the middle of my back, which is a bit unconventional to many people. But it fits me, as I live "imperfectly with great delight!"

GRAY8 TIPS & TECHNIQUES

I use Suave Coconut Conditioner, to wash and condition my hair. I also use a small dab of Desert Essence Soft Curls Hair Cream, Coconut, which I buy at the Health Food Market. I use Paul Mitchell Shampoo One every third shampoo to clarify my hair. Here are six great hair care tips:

1. Know your hair type and care for it accordingly.
2. Treat your hair gently; gray hair is fragile.
3. Avoid using heat on your hair; heat can turn gray hair yellow.
4. Keep your hair covered in the sun.
5. I have wavy hair, so I don't use a brush. I use either a wide-toothed comb or my fingers.
6. If you have wavy or curly hair, buy "Curly Girl The Handbook" by Lorraine Massey with Michele Bender—it works!

Lauren Traverson
Age 23
Missouri

I have always had a passion for helping animals and advocating for them, so it's no surprise that I work as a veterinary assistant. I am also currently a college student, trying to decide if I want to major in science or art, but I find myself leaning more towards the arts. I have been an artist for as long as I can remember and love to create, draw and paint. I also like to explore new places, travel, and go camping. I love to spend time with my family, and I enjoy reading anything and everything.

I started going gray when I was about thirteen or fourteen years old. Graying young is a common occurrence on my mother's side of the family. However, I am the youngest to go gray so far. Growing up, I had pitched-black hair and pale porcelain skin. When I started to go gray, it was a salt and pepper mixture, but as I have gotten older, it has become lighter and is more silver and white now.

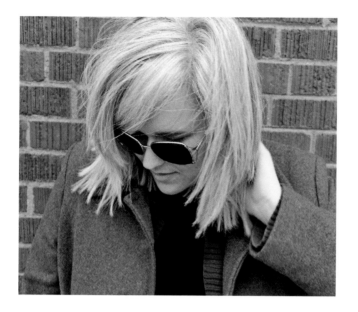

I remember being in the eighth grade and begging my mother to take me to the nearest store to buy hair dye to cover my gray hair. In a society that is obsessed with youth and staying young, going gray so early was very devastating. As a teenager in a small Midwestern town, all I wanted to do was, either fit in with the crowd or to be left alone. At that age, I felt as though having gray hair made me stand out too much, and made me a target to be potentially bullied. Sometimes children can be cruel just because you look different.

From that point on, until I was approximately 20-years-old, I dyed my hair different hues of browns and reds to cover the gray. Then, while attending college, it got to the point where I could no longer afford to dye my white roots every two weeks! Between not being able to afford the dye, and seeing how fried my hair was (from the chemicals in the dye), I decided to stop dyeing my hair and let my natural hair come in.

When I made the decision to go gray, I had no idea of the journey I was about to embark on. Although I had half-faded brown and red hair, I didn't have the gumption to cut it off, so I just let my hair grow and kept the ends trimmed. A few years later, when I had quite a bit of length, I decided to cut my hair. Now I am completely gray and dye-free. I love it!

Having gray hair has become a staple of my personality and is a regular conversation-starter. It has prompted people to approach me and ask questions about it, as well as brought me out of my shell of shyness. I have embraced my natural color and have cast all the beauty standards of this society to the wind.

Some of my peers don't understand as to why I would go this route. Why would I willingly choose to look much older than I am? For me, it is so much more than that. I feel like a genuine authentic person. Accepting my gray hair at such a young age has also allowed me to embrace and accept many other parts of myself. I feel that there is no better feeling in the world than when you can appreciate and love yourself for who you are. When you feel like the most authentic version of yourself, people around you will appreciate you for that. It will attract like-minded people.

It has not been an easy journey. I never imagined I would have a head full of gray hair at this age, but I honestly wouldn't trade it for the world.

GRAY8 TIPS & TECHNIQUES

My favorite hair care products are Paul Mitchell Tea Tree Lavender Mint Moisturizing Shampoo and Conditioner.

For those of you, who are considering embarking on the going gray journey, I encourage it whole-heartedly. It is not something that will be easy, by any means, but it is certainly well worth it! Today, you will find several groups online where others are making the same choices and are ready to support you in yours. Going gray has allowed me to be the most authentic version of me and is the best decision I have ever made. I not only wish the same feeling of love and acceptance to those making the journey, but to all of you on this beautiful earth. We only live once, so we might as well be as true to ourselves as we can. What do you have to lose?

Leesa Travis
Age 51
California

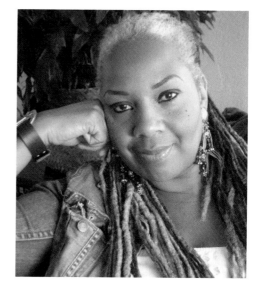

I am the youngest of five children, with three sisters and one brother. My parents were born and raised in Atlanta, Georgia, but moved to San Francisco before I was born. As a child, I grew up in a very strict house-hold. My father had certain guidelines and expected them to be followed. If they weren't, he would quickly remind us that we represented the Travis household. Needless to say, I spent most of my youth rebelling. I remember, when I was about nineteen, wearing my hair in a rebellious Mohawk!

As far back as I can remember, my father had beautiful white hair, but as a child I associated his white hair with being much older than my mother. So I was surprised to learn years later, that my parents were only a few years apart in age. I often teased my father about being such an old man, married to my much younger mother. I didn't realize that he had gone gray very young in life.

I always loved my father's white hair, and, as a teenager, I went out and bought a can of silver hair-spray so I could have beautiful white hair, too. My mother often told us that his gray hair was a Travis birthmark. My sister Adrienne also had the birthmark. She had jet-black hair with a gray patch right on top. When my sister and I would go out, I would grab my can of silver hairspray and start spraying.

People would often stop me and ask if that was really my hair, but before I could answer, my sister would interrupt, saying, "Hers is fake; mine is real!"

For years, my hair had always been a problem for me. Growing up as a young black child, it wasn't nappy enough to wear in an afro, and it wasn't straight enough to be called good hair. My hair was a soft, cotton-like mess. I would perm it, press it, curl it, braid it, and often choose to cut it very short, close to the scalp.

1994 was a hard year for me. I was a newly separated mother raising two sons and working as a makeup artist. During this time, I sported a short afro that was quick and easy to maintain. Then, in October, I visited my father, who had been ill for some time and was not doing well. I was glad to see my dad; we had patched up our differences years ago (after my first son was born), and he had grown to love my rebellious personality. As he lay there, I rubbed his soft, cotton-white hair and told him how much I loved him. When my sister Phyllis and I drove away, we knew we would not see him again. He died two days later. A couple weeks after my father's death, I noticed my hair had started to turn white just like my father's. It was exciting to see the gray hair come in. People associated it with stress, but I knew it was just a last gift from my dad.

Over the next three years, I wore my hair in many different styles. I loved my gray hair, but hated the texture, so, in 1997, I decided to shave my head and start over! I was determined to learn how to love my hair, not only the color, but also the texture and everything about it. I decided to grow dreadlocks.

Today I have long silver dreadlocks, but the very back of my hair is still all black. My hair looks and feels strong and regal, just like my father's. The best thing about my hair is that it is a complete reflection of who I am. I get stopped daily, (that is not an exaggeration) with compliments about my hair. The compliments never get old, because of how long it took for me to finally appreciate my hair. It's funny that I'm the youngest in my family and the only one who doesn't cover my gray. I guess I'm still a rebel!

GRAY8 TIPS & TECHNIQUES
To keep my White/Silver/Gray hair sparkling, I use Clairol Shimmer Lights, and I moisturize my dreadlocks with coconut oil.

Linda Love Atwater
Age 62
Arizona

I was a "talker" in school, and spent a lot of time in the hallway. I guess God decided I really needed to learn geography, so this California girl has spent most of her life moving. I have lived in California, Oregon, Washington, Arkansas, Michigan, New York, Maryland, Texas, Florida, Nebraska, Arizona, and Massachusetts.

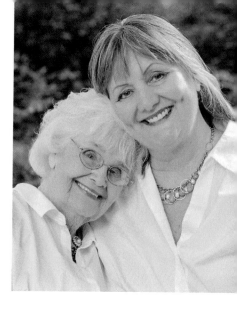

I was married at nineteen, had two children, got a divorce, and later remarried. I managed banks and credit unions, worked in nuclear power plants, and currently own my own business as a professional organizer. At the tender age of three, I would go to my aunt's house and organize her canned goods in the cabinet. So as you can see, my organizing days go way back!

My mother is 88, but don't tell her I told you. I don't remember ever seeing her natural hair color until she quit coloring just a few years ago. I would help her color her roots from a very young age. I remember the gloves, the mixing, the shaking, and the smell. I thought everyone had special towels with dye stains that were used for this (every few week) event. I don't know if you would call it a mother-daughter bonding experience, but it opened the door to my dye addiction.

When I was sixteen, I began my "Lets cover what Mother Nature gave me" campaign, and continued coloring until I was 55-years-old. I started with "Sun In," since it was the 60's and the magazines told us that blonde was the cool look. Since then, my hair has been blonde, red, highlighted, low lighted, and, once (by accident), Bart Simpson orange! Add in the perms, cuts, and conditioning, and I spent a fortune on my hair. Once I quit work, I decided it was time to quit wearing the work clothes, the heels, and the makeup. One day, I was glancing through a catalog and noticed this beautiful model with natural gray hair. I ripped out that page and said to myself, "This is what I want!"

I really don't have a gray8 hair story; I just decided one day that I was done coloring my hair, spending the money, and finding a stylist every time we moved. At the time, we were living in Florida. As a hair dye addict, I found it scarier to find a stylist (every time we moved), than it was, to find a doctor for my yearly OBGYN! At my next hair appointment, I handed the stylist my ripped-out page and said, "I am going to grow my hair out and look like this." I know she saw dollar bills fly out of her future and replied, "You don't want to do that; you'll look old." I insisted that I did, and, with a deep sigh, she said, "Okay, let's cut it in layers and put highlights on the roots." And, with that, my journey to gray had started.

My hair has never looked or felt better. I did not get the pretty silver/white hair of my mother. I got the salt and pepper hair of my father. I love looking through my hair and seeing the different colors that Mother Nature gave me: silver, brown, red, and black, and how they work perfectly with my blue eyes and complexion. If you are like me, you will notice that, as your hair becomes authentic, other parts of your life will, too. Enjoy your journey, and find comfort in the fact that you will never put chemicals on your head again, and that you have many silver sisters standing beside you in spirit!

GRAY8 TIPS & TECHNIQUES

My hair is like horse hair! LOL! It is very coarse, thick, straight, healthy, and shiny. I can curl it, but the curl falls out with just the slightest bit of humidity. I use baby shampoo, but do not use any type of conditioner after shampooing and let it dry naturally. If I feel a product build-up on my hair, I use a white vinegar and water rinse. Once or twice a month I use a purple shampoo. I use extra-virgin coconut oil as a deep-conditioner and leave it in 20 to 30 minutes, then wash my hair. I have my hair trimmed about every couple of months, unless it gets too wild and crazy; and then I will go ahead and have it cut sooner.

One thing I noticed with my natural hair is that, I needed to change out some of my wardrobe colors. The beige and brown tones that looked great on me as a blonde, no longer looked good on me. Now I wear jewel-tone colors along with neutral shades like gray, black, and white.

As a professional organizer, I suggest that you put a garbage bag in your closet, and when you try on an item that doesn't look or feel right, fold it up and put it in the bag. Pass those blessings onto others. Put your hangers with the hooks facing towards you. When you wear an item and put it back in the closet, turn the hanger around. At the end of the year or season, you will know which clothes you wear the most and which ones you can pass on.

Photo credit: Ingrid Hunsicker Photography

Lois Khalafalla
Age 48
North Carolina

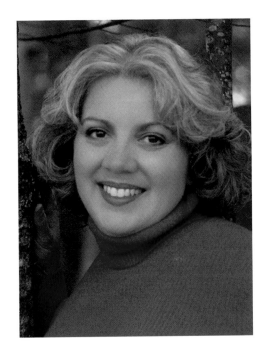

When I first started seeing gray hairs in my 20's, I automatically thought I needed to dye my hair. It just seemed like the natural thing to do. I didn't do it that often, and it really did not interfere with anything in my life. But, as the years continued, I found myself dyeing my hair more often, at least once a month. Then, around age 44, I was coloring my hair every three weeks to keep my roots under control. My husband had urged me to stop dyeing for years. No way! Maybe in my 60's, I said.

Eventually, I grew tired of the routine and gave going natural a try. I had about three inches of growth, when one day, someone made a bad comment about my hair. That one comment sent me back to dyeing my hair for another year; it was horrible. At this point, I now was getting only two good weeks out of each color session before the gray started showing again. My hair was turning to straw and falling out! My hair would actually crunch when I put it in a ponytail. Plus, I had people commenting on how thin my hair had become.

My husband continued to urge me to stop the madness! So, I did some research on the Internet and found many support groups. I was amazed that I was not alone. There were so many beautiful women with silver, white, and gray hair! Reading their stories was so inspiring to me. I then decided I've had enough! So I stopped dyeing my hair.

About six weeks in, I had about one inch of new growth, and I couldn't take my ugly, crunching, dyed hair anymore, so I buzzed it! My husband encouraged me to go ahead and start fresh. He really is wonderful. My children, on the other hand, were a different story. I have six children, five boys and one girl. Their ages are (26), (21), (16), (15), (10), and (8). My daughter was especially upset. Everyone always told us she looked just like me. She was so afraid we wouldn't look alike anymore.

It was a hard decision, but I felt if I didn't start fresh, I would give in and dye my hair again. I took out the clippers one morning and started buzzing (down to three-quarters of an inch)! When my husband saw me, he told me how beautiful I was! My boys said I looked strange, and they didn't like it, and my daughter cried, (oh, boy, that was hard). I tried to explain to her that I had to be true to myself. I got impolite comments from some people, but for the most part, people were very encouraging. I took a picture each month for one year.

It was amazing watching my new, soft multicolored hair grow. It had natural highlights. I couldn't keep my hands out of my hair. It was so soft! I felt empowered! I had taken control of my life. I know— you are probably thinking, how is NOT dyeing your hair taking control? But it is! It really is. It changes you inside and out. I didn't have to do what society said I should do. I was free! My hair continued to grow, and there were some hard stages to go through.

I will never forget the day my daughter and I were shopping, and the cashier said, "Your daughter looks just like you!" I turned to my daughter, and I just smiled. She was smiling, too. Gray hair hadn't taken away from our similarities, after all! Now, when my children see an old picture of me, they say that I looked weird. My daughter now makes avatars with gray hair. She tells me she thinks my hair is pretty. I love it. I wouldn't change a thing. I love being dye-free. I love not having roots. I love not having to plan my life around when I will dye my hair. I am free to live carefree! At least when it comes to my hair!

GRAY8 TIPS & TECHNIQUES
I use Pantene Pro-V Silver Expressions to keep my silvers nice and bright.

If you decide you want to transition to gray, be confident in your decision, and don't let others try to sway you into doing what "they" think you should do. If you decide you want to continue dyeing your hair, that's okay, too. Always make the decision that works best for you.

Lori Murray

Age 52

New York

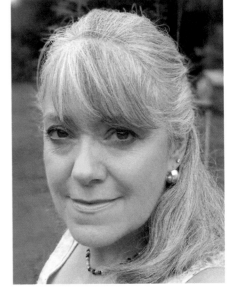

On December 30th, 2011, I decided, that this would be the last time I colored my hair. In the months prior to this decision, I had been really contemplating it. When my regrowth would begin to show, I would pull all my hair back, so I could only see the gray. And finally I thought, "Why not?" I was 50-years-old and had been coloring my hair for several decades.

I began my going gray journey by purchasing a few silver/gray wigs that I thought would be close to my (now) natural hair color. This really gave me a feel for how I would look in gray hair. It also helped me to know for sure, if I was ready to transition. The dye had been irritating my scalp for the past couple years, leaving me with little blisters that would take up to a couple weeks to heal, each time I colored.

I had been wearing my hair quite long and really dreaded the idea of two-tone hair for several years. My husband really likes my long hair, and supported the natural color transition. I told him I was going to grow it for six months, then cut it all off, and he would just have to deal with it. I wasn't going to nurse it along slowly, trimming the color away little by little. He wasn't happy at the prospect of a short-haired me, but once late June 2012 rolled around, that's just exactly what I did. I got a pixie cut, and personally I really enjoyed the change. Of course, my other half did not! So, here I am a year-and-a-half later, still growing it out. I have a few inches to go, but I have enjoyed it every step of the way. I like it long, and I liked it short!

I get more compliments than I ever did before. People often ask me if my color is natural. It's not uncommon for a total stranger to compliment my hair in passing. And, if you enjoy your hair long, you can certainly wear it long! Somehow, our society has conditioned women to think they can't wear long hair after 40, but that's just not true!

Incidentally, I have been a hairdresser for over 30 years, and, naturally, I support any client who chooses to go gray. Allowing your hair to go natural is a personal decision. Don't let anyone else make the decision for you. I hate to see my clients, who have decided to give it a try, get negative feedback from friends and family, but it does happen. What is everyone afraid of? If you're ready, don't let that discourage you; just go for it. I believe that most often Mother Nature knows best. As our faces age, a softer color framing us is generally more complementary to our features. Your own natural gray, silver, or salt and pepper hair is uniquely yours! So let your SILVER-LOCKS-ROCK!

I grew up in the southern tier of New York State, along with a sister and three brothers. I met my husband James, later in life, and we have been together now for ten years. We both enjoy gardening, boating, hiking, and camping.

GRAY8 TIPS & TECHNIQUES

Buying a wig really helped me during my transition. I could see what I might look like with gray hair and adjust to it mentally. At the same time, it also helped cover the demarcation line. I picked a style I was very comfortable with, and one that would be easy to work with. Find a hairdresser that will work with you during your transition. You will need someone who is supportive and will work with you to make your transition easier. Don't let anyone, even your hairdresser; tell you that you "should" color your hair. Adding in some very pale to silver highlights through your hair, can help ease the transition—but understand that it will not replicate your unique shade. However, it can help take the edge off as you grow your hair out.

Lynn C.
Age 54
Alaska

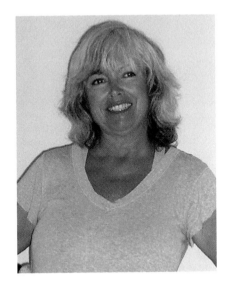

A couple of years ago, I lost my most beloved horse of fourteen years, and the loss was so traumatic for me that, at that very moment, I decided to make a complete life change. I retired from my job of ten years, decided to relocate back home to Alaska permanently, and I also decided to go completely natural with my hair color (which is and always has been a gorgeous silvery color).

I started showing the silvers when I was in my mid-20's, and, of course, a woman back then "would" never, "should" never, let her hair go gray! For the life of me, I still cannot believe that I fell for all that malarkey, but I did, and I dyed my hair for over 25 years.

When I decided to be free of the dye, my hair was booty-length. I am one of those "all or nothing" kind of girls, so there was no way I was going to have two-tone hair; therefore, I chopped my hair into a pixie cut. I just looked in the mirror, took my scissors out—and cut! Nope, no hair cutting experience for this girl. I just thought, how could I go wrong? I wanted to make the transition quick, and I did! I was so elated!

I felt free, healthy, and more vibrant than ever. Oh sure, there were some that thought I had lost my marbles, but I didn't care. I was committed, I knew what I wanted and why, and I have never looked back since. My silver hair is soft and healthy. My scalp no longer has that horrible scaly stuff on it and I no longer put chemicals on my brain. And guess what? It's just plain prettier! My hair matches my skin tone, just as Mother Nature intended.

I have cut my hair three times since I went natural. Sometimes, I think I want my hair long, but lately, I'm thinking of a pixie again! Since going natural, I have had more compliments on my hair than I have ever had. Women come up to me and say, "I wish I had the courage to go natural." Yep, it takes confidence to be silver, no doubt, and it shows, and it's sexy! SILVER ROCKS!

I am a mom, a grandmother, and an equestrian, and I live every day like it's my last!

GRAY8 TIPS & TECHNIQUES

I use only organic, all-natural products on my hair. My favorite go-to hair product is Aveda Blue Malva Shampoo and Conditioner. I use organic coconut oil as a leave-in and also as a deep-conditioner. I cut my own bangs, and currently I am letting my hair grow long.

For makeup, I can now wear pinks and reds. For wardrobe, I look great in black, white, and gray.

Marina Capello
Age 50
Italy

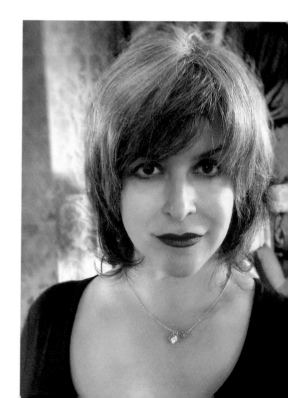

I was born and raised in Italy and enjoy travelling, reading, good food, metaphysics, fashion, singing and trekking.

I stopped dyeing my hair in 2005, but started thinking about it a year prior when I was in Las Vegas. I saw a lady working in Neman Marcus, and was struck by the beauty of her salt and pepper hair and funky haircut. I told her, "One day, I will do the same as you," but I knew I wasn't ready yet.

In 2004, I was wearing my hair medium-length, straight, and dyeing it dark brown; my natural colour was nearly black. By this time, I had been dyeing my hair for nearly a decade and had no clue as to how much white I actually had.

Then, one fine day, I was looking through the pages of a French "Elle" Magazine. I noticed a young female model with grey hair. She looked fantastic, and her hair colour was so different from anyone else's. I loved it! That was the turning point in my decision to grow out my natural hair colour. I was afraid but curious to see what was underneath all the dye and what my natural hair would look like. But although I was really excited, not everyone around me was. I was completely unsupported by all of my family and peers. During my transition, I searched the Internet for inspiring, beautiful grey-haired ladies, and got my strength from there.

I let my hair grow for about three months, wearing it pulled back into a ponytail. Then, I decided to go cold turkey and had it cut short! I live close to London, so it is very easy to find a salon to do a superb funky cut! I got it done just like the lady I saw in Vegas. What a change that was! I can safely say by month seven, I was rid of any colour. I continued to wear my hair short for a while and then decided to let it grow. My hair grows very fast, so it wasn't long before it was below my collar bone. I love my hair, and it is a lot more shiny and thick now, whereas when I was dyeing my hair, it was limp and dull, except for the first couple of weeks of new colouring!

I work as a PR consultant, organizing big events, and I'm often involved in the fashion and beauty industry. Appearances are very important to what I do. Keeping groomed and glamorous has helped me in the process. I realise now, after a decade of colouring, that the colour of one's hair does not really matter and does not age you. It is our vibrancy and vitality that determines how people perceive us.

I had a few ladies who thanked me for inspiring them to go natural, which made me so happy, as I was inspired myself to be different from the rest of the crowd. I am chemical-free and never have to worry again about my roots on a windy day! It was not easy, but I am so thrilled I did it and will not look back.

Any hostility and criticism I received came from women, not men. In fact, men seem to find my salt and pepper hair very sexy. Going natural is not for everybody, but if you want to honor what Mother Nature has in store for you, then it's for you! Now, I am asked if I dye my hair to make it look this way!

My face still looks young, which makes an unusual contrast to my salt and pepper hair. And, last but not least, when I was recently on holiday visiting my mum, she said, "You were right in being stubborn about your hair; it looks superb now." Phew! My mum was the one who had resisted my decision the most!

I don't believe the colour of a woman's hair ages her at all. It is a mixture of many things that can age a person. I choose to see beauty and positivity in all that surrounds me. I love my life, and, yes, I love my grey hair, too!

GRAY8 TIPS & TECHNIQUES

I switch between Klorane Shampoo with Magnolia and Kerastase Bain Chroma Riche. For style, my favorite product is Aveda Control Paste.

My best advice for anyone going grey is to always keep yourself well-groomed. An up-to-date, edgy haircut always works wonders. Exercise; taking brisk walks, will help keep your figure trim. And, to keep your skin glowing, avoid the sun, and drink plenty of water, and, of course, wear red lipstick!

Melissa Dickson Fleury
Age 41
Arizona

I am an active mother with two young children ages three and five, and I spend my mornings like many other moms with young kiddos. I try to cram in every little errand or project I can before picking the kids up from school. Then I spend the rest of the day chasing after them, and trying to maintain my sanity.

I love to spend my time running. I run several times a week and just completed my second half-marathon. I plan to run a full marathon within the next year or two. A few years ago, I started a local running group that is specifically for moms. We're now up to over 100 women, and range in ages from the 30's to the 40's. I'm not the youngest in my group, but I AM the only one with gray hair! Gasp!

I stopped coloring my hair when I was 39, and I truly feel it was one of the best decisions I have ever made. When I pick up the kids at school, I'm the only mommy with gray hair. Standing out in this way originally scared the crap out of me; I didn't want people to think I was my kids' grandma. Now, I like the fact that I look unique, and not like the sea of other women, with long colored hair.

When I decided to go gray, I did a little bit of everything during my transition. I had been previously highlighting my hair, in an attempt to hide the gray, and so my overall hair color, was much lighter than my natural pigmented hair. So, the first thing I did was have my stylist dye my hair, (avoiding new growth) so that the line of demarcation would be less severe. At about two or three months into my grow-out, I decided to have some highlights put in around my face and regretted it almost immediately. If I had it to do over again, I'd skip that step! At that point, I quit coloring cold turkey. I let my gray hair grow out for eight months, and then chopped off the remaining cosmetic color, after months of agonizing over whether or not to cut it! LOL! The initial shock of having hair that was suddenly SHORT AND GRAY was pretty overwhelming. This process is about so much more than hair color. It has been an amazing journey of self-acceptance and self-confidence.

I have been absolutely floored by the constant compliments and comments I get from women every single day! "Your hair is amazing!" "I would absolutely stop coloring my hair if my gray looked like yours!" The thing is, their gray is most likely just as fabulous, but they'll never know! They're so tightly gripped by fear that they won't ever take the leap to find out what wonderful and completely unique shade of gray/white/silver they might possess.

It does feel like a leap when you decide to stop coloring your hair, a leap right off a cliff! Making the choice to stop coloring your hair is a scary one. Everyone around you will be full of opinions and advice. Not all of it will be helpful or kind. Just try to remember that most of that advice comes from a place of fear, fear of aging, fear of no longer looking attractive or sexy, fear that suddenly everyone won't think you're 25 verses 40 anymore etc. News flash! Nobody thinks you're 25, anyway!

Here is my two cents on the topic of gray hair: I believe progress is being made. I'm seeing more beauty, fashion, clothing, websites now listing their Photoshop Policy, stating that they don't re-touch the photos of their models, and some use women that aren't models by profession, but rather every day women, who work for their company. They state that each woman has her own unique beauty and that this isn't something that should be corrected or changed. Let's hope the winds of change are blowing! It will hopefully be easier for this generation to also embrace their true unique beauty as they age, when they aren't bombarded with unrealistic images of women spending endless amounts of time and money in the pursuit of looking younger.

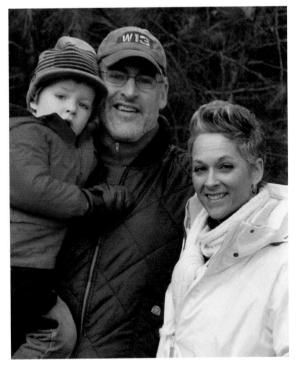

There is already a bit of a movement underway today! There are many women, who, like me, choose to take our authenticity even one step further by not coloring our hair. What could be more authentic and daring than that? Just because I don't color my hair, doesn't mean that I've let myself go; it doesn't mean that I don't want to look hip, or that I have no interest in fashion. There is a terrible misconception that going gray, equals letting yourself go, looking old, or just plain giving up. This couldn't be farther from the truth!

I have to wonder, if there were more women, like myself (relatively young and gray!) featured in magazines, on TV commercials, and on sitcoms, would more women feel confident in their own unique beauty to truly embrace their authentic self, gray hair and all? I am a member of several groups full of women from all over the world, who are embracing their natural beauty. When you stop coloring, you're not only changing your outward appearance, but there is also an internal transformation that takes place, when you decide to fly in the face of societal norms and stop this futile attempt to look younger. For me, it started with, "What is so wrong with looking my age, anyway?" People have a completely false/skewed view of what forty looks like, anyway, because EVERYONE colors their hair these days. They wouldn't know what forty looked like even if it jumped up and bit them in the A$$! Then I felt inspired, in an admittedly that's total BS (I'll show them) kind of way. You have to realize that hair color doesn't make you look younger. I wasn't fooling anyone, and why on earth would I want to, anyway?

Having gray hair doesn't have to mean old or letting yourself go. You can still be the same fun, active, silly person you've always been!

GRAY8 TIPS & TECHNIQUES

Some of my favorite hair products include: Shea Moisture Coconut and Hibiscus Curl and Style Milk for thick curly hair. I also use either Organix Repairing Awapuhi Ginger Dry Styling Oil or MOROC-CANOIL Treatment Light.

Your hair does not define you! Looking younger doesn't make you more attractive, and it certainly won't make you happy. What we should be after is self-acceptance, which then leads to self-confidence, and nothing is sexier than self-confidence! I'd love to see more women take this journey, and hopefully the numbers will continue to grow, as gray support groups become more well-known. Embracing your authentic self is a wonderful experience, and; what could be a better lesson to teach our children?

Michelle Burge
Age 50
Ohio

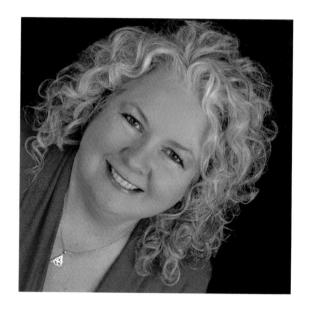

I am one of seven children, third from the last and the quiet one. I married my high school sweetheart right after I graduated high school and have two amazing children. I was married for eleven years, but, as we grew up, we grew apart. As a single mother, I was working full-time as a secretary. But my dream was to have my own business someday, so, as a single mom in my 30's; I made it happen and opened my own video store, where you can still find me fourteen years later. Now I am married to my best friend and the love of my life, with two beautiful granddaughters. I have learned to believe that life is what you make it!

I was one of those women who said, "I will never let my hair go gray." Well, look at me now; I have wild and crazy silver-gray curls, and I love them! When I said I would never go gray, I really did believe it at the time. Not that I didn't have plenty of gray hairs, because I did. You just couldn't see them under all that hair dye. What started out as an every two month process at age 25, turned out to be an every three week process by the time I was 42, (with a touch of brown mascara) to hold me over between salon visits. I even remember getting sores on the back of my head from coloring, but still could not stop. For some reason, I just kept thinking I was too young and that gray hair would make me look too old. It just never occurred to me that not coloring was an option. I lived and scheduled every event in my life around coloring my hair.

Then, at 42, my health drastically changed. I was diagnosed with uterine cancer. The next four years proved to be a challenge. After my last surgery, I ended up with complications that would last six months. Now, going to the salon was nearly impossible, but somehow I managed to color a couple more times. Having health issues really puts things into perspective. I started thinking about my life and what was important and what was not. As I lay in bed one morning, needing my roots done again, I thought, why not let my hair go gray and see what I think? So I got on my computer and searched going gray! I was amazed that I found so many women out there with beautiful gray hair. I read every story that I could find and looked at every picture. They not only had beautiful gray hair, but they didn't look old and seemed happy, healthy, and confident! But how could that be? They let their hair go gray. Well, that's all it took for me, and I have never looked back since. I knew then that I wanted my natural silver to shine, too! At first, I was worried my curls would go away, but, as you can see, they are still there! My hair is softer and healthier than it has ever been, and, yes, it's gray!

Going gray was not always an easy journey for me, but it was one that I loved in so many ways. It has transformed me into the woman that I am today and have always wanted to be; I love being me! If you decide to go gray, do it with your head held high, and enjoy the journey to your authentic happy self!

When I look back, I realize that not everyone was on board with my decision. My daughter thought I was letting myself go and that I would look younger if I colored. But that statement is the farthest thing from the truth! She has learned to accept and kind of like, my silver-gray curls now, and my husband says he could not imagine me any other way. It has been over a year now since my last surgery, after which I spent four days in intensive care fighting for my life. Cancer changes you as a person; I have so much to be thankful for, and every day, I look forward to the rest of my life.

GRAY8 TIPS & TECHNIQUES

I wash my hair almost every day and use DevaCurl Hair Products. I shampoo with DevaCurl No-Poo and use One Conditioner. To define my curls, I use DevaCurl Light Defining Gel. A couple times a month, I use DevaCurl Heaven In Hair to deep-condition. Every five to six weeks, I add a small amount of baking soda to my shampoo and rinse with white vinegar, mixed with water. I have well water with iron, so baking soda keeps the yellow from building up in my hair. I apply the gel for styling and blow-dry with a diffuser attachment while my head is tilted down.

Monica Gallacher

Age 45

Massachusetts

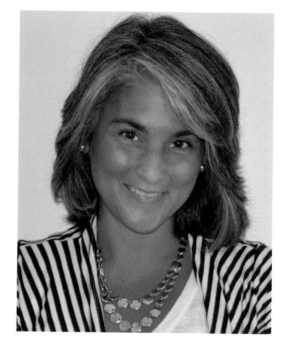

Having grown up in New Jersey in the 70's and 80's, I know all about good hair. By ethnicity, I'm Italian, Peruvian, Spanish, and Danish, and my hair was naturally very dark brown (almost black) and poker-straight, with lots of shine and volume. It was the one physical attribute that made me feel special, and I can honestly say, I appreciated it, and have always taken good care of my locks. I got regular trims, (every six to eight weeks), since my teens, and have always used good quality hair products.

The grays started cropping up in my early 20's, and at the time, I liked the novelty of them. I thought I would just watch with amazement as a fabulous silver streak emerged in the front of my hair and I'd rock that look like Anne Bancroft in "The Graduate" or Alexandra from "Josie and the Pussycats." But instead, I had wiry gray hairs scattered throughout, so I started single-process coloring, in my early 30's. After a decade of doing that, I began refreshing my roots every fourteen to eighteen days with do-it-yourself at-home coloring kits, to save money and time. The color no longer looked natural, and the maintenance was tedious.

Going silver was always a goal of mine; however, I always figured it would happen in my 50's or 60's. But surprisingly, my epiphany came when my oldest daughter entered high school. I had a vision of sending her off to college someday, and being "that" mom with the bad dye job. That's when it struck me, that it was time to stop pretending that I was still a brunette, and find out exactly what was underneath all that dye. After some tears and trepidation about aging too quickly, I embarked on the journey one year ago. I had the support of my very cool husband (who's been with me for 25 years) and our two surprisingly diplomatic teenaged daughters. So with the guidance of my trusted stylist/colorist, I started my journey.

After discussing several options, including going cold turkey or getting a pixie cut, I opted for heavy highlights. Following three weeks of not coloring, there was enough growth for my stylist to figure out a plan. In the front I was about 85 percent gray, fading to about 25 percent in the back and underneath. Since I had such processed hair, my colorist could only go with blonde highlights (rather than silver) to help camouflage the inevitable skunk stripe and ease the transition. The highlights were done in June 2014 and again in late August to lighten the blonde even more. Lowlights of warmer brown were added in October to tone things down a bit, and the lighter areas were made more platinum.

In the beginning my hair was a combination of blonde, medium brown, silver, and dark brown. For me, it was definitely the right way to transition; I wasn't courageous enough to let the skunk stripe show, nor did I have the confidence to rock a pixie. As far as length, I usually have shoulder-length hair with layers and long bangs, but I opted to go shorter during my transition to lose some of the darker hair. It was okay, but will definitely grow it long again. That's just how I feel most comfortable.

During the early stages of my transition, I definitely indulged in a bit of self-pity, feeling that the days of my youth were behind me, and that I'd lost that unique piece of my physical identity. I have learned that the journey of "un-wrapping the silver" is more about self-discovery and seeking authenticity, than it is about the color of my hair. Underneath the surface, it's all about being comfortable in your own skin, and, if that means going "au natural," fantastic. If it means choosing to color, that's fabulous too. It's simply being content in the present moment and seeing and loving the beauty inside and not needing external praise.

As a mom determined to raise happy, confident, well-adjusted daughters, I honestly feel that beauty isn't about the color of our hair or any other physical attribute; it's about knowing and loving ourselves for all the goodness that resides in our hearts and radiates outward. My older sister (who has yet to get a single gray hair) shared this Bible verse, which has been very empowering: "Gray hair is a crown of splendor; it is attained in the ways of righteousness." Proverbs 16:31.

To date, each strand of gray hair holds part of my life story, and the new ones that emerge, will follow suit. I'm finally ready to re-read the old chapters of my life and for the rest to be written, "one silver strand at a time." And, for the record, even though I've lived in Massachusetts for fifteen years, I still have pretty good New Jersey hair!

I'm nearly finished with my transition, with about one inch of highlights left on the ends. It's been a liberating experience. As a trusted friend always reminded me, "It's just hair; you can always change it, if you don't like it!"

GRAY8 TIPS & TECHNIQUES

My current favorite hair care lines are Kevin Murphy, Living Proof, and Alterna Caviar.

For inspiration I started a Pinterest board with photos of beautiful silver-haired women. I also follow pages on Facebook that empower women choosing to go gray. This has helped me stay focused and enthusiastic during my transition.

Monica Ludwig

Age 50

Virginia

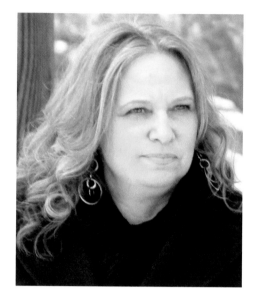

I was born in Baltimore, Maryland, and grew up in a blue-collar town, where my dad was a steelworker. He hated his job, and education was top priority in our house. I grew up with three older brothers, and we all went on to college and earned advanced degrees. I have a BS in Elementary Education, and a Master's in Education as well. I taught many years in the public school system and then became a Reading Specialist. In 1989, I met my husband Bill, and we married in 1993. Then, in 1996, we started our family and now have four children: Addison, Dane, Ainsley, and Sage. My life has been very busy with this big brood, but I feel incredibly blessed every day. I currently work as an online professor for American Public University, and I am also a consultant for a health and wellness company.

There were a series of events that prompted me to want to ditch the dye. First of all, for many years, I only highlighted my hair. This was a wonderful thing while it lasted. However, my gray hair was coming in fast and furious, and I started to do all-over color when I was about 37. During the next ten years, I religiously colored my hair every six weeks or so. Slowly but surely, I noticed that my hair was becoming thinner. By the time I turned 47, my scalp clearly started to develop a sensitivity to the dye. Having thin hair with an irritated scalp was not fun, for sure.

However, I think the catalyst that put me over the edge was when I was at Home Depot. Yes, the Home Depot! A woman was working there who had a long mane of silver hair. It was amazing! She shared her story, and it was freakishly comparable to mine. That was it! I stopped dyeing my hair in June 2011. I let it grow for eleven months and had it cut into a long pixie. My goal is whatever length I can get, while still maintaining my hair's health. It has been an interesting journey, but one I would not change. I finally feel authentic!

As far as support, my husband has been my biggest fan. We are now a matching set! Quite honestly, I have not received any negative feedback from others. I have gotten many compliments, and most people think my hair is frosted! I still have a fair amount of my natural brown mixed in. I just love all the mélange of colors!

GRAY8 TIPS & TECHNIQUES

Since I have very fine, wavy hair, I need to treat my hair like silk. I use sulfate-free Alba Botanical Natural Hawaiian Shampoo, and, truth be told, my favorite silicone-free conditioner is Suave Conditioner (under two bucks); it's the best! I use a twelve minute heavy-duty deep-conditioner, once a month by George Michael Long Hair Products (they specialize in long hair care). And I get a long hair treatment every six weeks from the George Michael Salon. I get my hair trimmed every four months to keep it healthy. I really don't use anything for the gray since it has not yellowed.

Natalie Benton
Age 55
Kansas

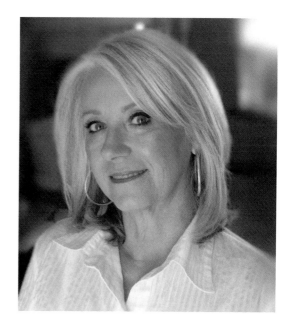

My story is not unlike the stories of many other beautiful women who have made the transition to silver. Let me start by telling you a little about me. I am "that" girl who was a high school cheerleader, hid makeup from her mother, and applied it as soon as she got on the school bus. I am infamous for my laugh, the fact that I know the name of almost every MAC eye shadow color, and that I never leave the house without my face-on! I got married young and divorced six months after my beautiful daughter was born. I was a single mom for thirteen years, enjoying our girl-time and never thinking I needed a man in my life. Suddenly, out of the blue, along comes my high school sweetheart, my first love. We hadn't seen each other in 22 years, and it was love at first sight. We were engaged within two months after our first date, and have now been joyfully married for fifteen years.

I struggle to find the words to explain the emotional part of my going gray journey. After my mother was diagnosed with cancer, she stayed with my husband and me. She loved for me to be present in the room with her every night, so—we started watching YouTube videos and talking about hair and makeup. When I was a little girl, I loved watching my mom do her hair and apply her makeup. I decided a few years ago to start making videos; it was a new way for mom and me to focus on something other than the cancer and treatment. We spoke often of how she had no gray hair at 70-years-old, and how my father was completely white by the time he was in his 40's. At this point, I was keenly aware that my hair was going to be just like daddy's. But there was NO WAY this girl was going gray!

I fought the gray, just as hard as mom fought cancer. Finding the time to go to the hairdresser's every four to five weeks for touch-ups, was starting to be a struggle. Mom needed me! She was in and out of the hospital so many times, and I spent hours caring for her. At some point, I just made the decision that there were too many more important things in life, than coloring my hair. My husband was encouraging me; he loved the idea of me going gray. During my transition I had my hairdresser start going lighter when she did my weave. We then started to use the silver as my highlights, and added some lowlights. Eventually, we just stopped coloring all together, so my transition was very subtle.

I feel we often learn things in our lives, which we don't realize at the time, until we look back. I don't think I knew until now, that was happening to me, as I watched mom suffer so terribly at the end of her life. She loved my new silver hair! She would encourage me, in her own way, suggesting I use a brighter lipstick, or more blush. I would walk into her room at the hospital, and I could feel her checking me out. I didn't mind, really; my transition was giving mom something else to focus on—and that was good.

Until I was asked to contribute to this book, I don't think I even knew that not only did I spend years saying goodbye to mom, but I also let go of my youthful way of thinking; that the color of my hair was important to who I was as a person. I am Natalie, a wife, mother, nana, sister, aunt, niece, friend, and SILVER!

PS: GOING GRAY ONCE AGAIN

In November of 2013, I went for my annual mammogram. The results were mailed to me, as they always are, stating that everything was fine. Then, on January 12, 2014, during a self-exam, I found a lump in my left breast. After several tests and biopsies, I was diagnosed with Stage 2, Triple Negative Invasive Ductal Cancer. On February 7, 2014, I received the first of what would be eight chemotherapy treatments. My oncologist said that my hair would start to fall out after my second treatment, so I chose to have my head shaved right away. I remember having a sense of urgency; I didn't want to wait until it started to fall out. I knew this was going to be a fight, and I wanted this cancer to know it had picked the wrong silver sister! My family participated in the "shaving;" we drank champagne, and a videographer captured my granddaughter taking the clippers to my hair. We all celebrated life and love, as my silver hair fell to the floor.

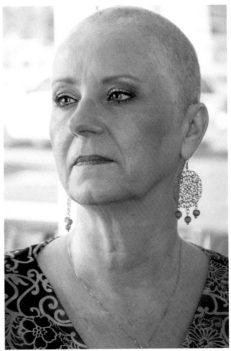

I have now completed chemotherapy, as well as surgery to remove the lump. Next stop: six weeks of daily radiation. There was no indication of cancer in my lymph nodes, my margins were clear, and my oncologist feels that I have had a complete response to chemotherapy.

My silver is growing back, and I could not be more proud of it! Please do not forget to check your "bumps for lumps!" Mammograms are so important, but they are NOT 100 percent accurate.

GRAY8 TIPS & TECHNIQUES

I use White Hot Hair Brilliant Shampoo (violet) once a week for yellowing, and use ColorProof Detox Shampoo for clarifying once a week to remove product build-up.

Patsy Telpner
Age 62
Canada

I lost my mother when I was 25. She was only 49-years-old. When I look back, I remember watching my mother colour her hair. She applied the colour leaving in a streak of grey hair. For years that streak of grey hair was an image I just couldn't shake. I didn't want that grey, and, in my case, it was so much more than just a grey streak.

I was 35 when I first started colouring my hair. I had grey hair sprouting from my forehead to the crown of my head. This was in 1987; I was living in Winnipeg, with two children ages eleven and nine, managing the household, and enjoying a very full life. I thought I was way too young to show any grey hair, and there was no way I would let it go grey.

I found colouring to be messy, costly, and time consuming. Sometimes the colour came out darker, and because of that, it made my grey roots stand out even more. There didn't seem to be a way out of this tiresome and expensive routine. In between colourings, I would touch-up the roots myself, making a mess of numerous towels and bathrobes.

My husband, whose hair was grey since his 30's, often, suggested that I should just let my hair go grey. He encouraged me, telling me that I would look great with grey hair, and I know he meant it. My response was, "I am not ready yet; maybe when I turn 60."

I have been a ceramic artist since my 20's, but, for the last few years, I have been focused on painting. During those 35 years as a potter, making functional work, I met numerous artists who let their hair go naturally grey. But I still was not convinced.

When I turned 59, I was the victim of a really bad haircut and an even worse hair colour. At the same time, my husband was diagnosed with prostate cancer. My daughter Meghan was a practicing holistic nutritionist, and advised me often that the dye I was putting onto my scalp was seriously toxic. In fact, it was carcinogenic.

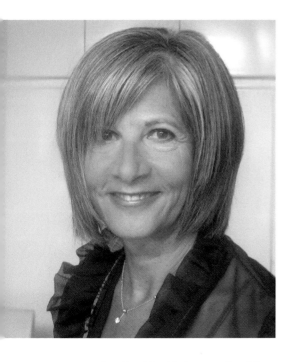

The final straw came when I was at an annual event, with artists from all over the city. I was chatting with a woman who had the most amazing grey hair. I began asking her questions about why she decided to go grey etc. Her response? "I had brain cancer, and I have no doubt that it was caused by the hair dye I had been using for so many years." That was all I needed to hear; I made up my mind, I was going to go grey!

I had been going to a beauty school for years for my hair, and became friends with an instructor named Grace; a very talented hair stylist. She would be my guide through this transition. She started by lightning my hair. At the time, my hair was almost black and looked very unnatural. It made me realize, that older women should not have black hair, or red hair, or orange hair, or any of the other unnatural-looking hair colour, that we often see women sporting. Once the cut was right, she put in a temporary rinse to blend in the grey, until it looked quite natural. I should add that much of the process occurred over the winter months, and living in a cold city, and wearing a hat from time to time, was very helpful in camouflaging the grey. It took about a year to transition and grow-out a bad haircut, but now I have the best hair ever!

I believe you should not sport grey hair that is long and untidy; it only ages you and makes you look as though you are living in the past. Believe me; a great haircut makes all the difference in the world. Not a day goes by that someone doesn't compliment me on my hair. And, because of a great hairstyle, I am often asked if I had my hair professionally streaked. Going grey has been great!

The strangest comment I get is, "You are so brave to go grey." That floors me! Brave? Hardly! There are so many people in the world who are brave, who fight every day for their country, religious beliefs, or to feed their families. Growing out your hair and leaving the dye off your scalp is smart, not brave.

As I write this, my husband and I are retired, although he still takes on selected clients. We have a house in the city and another in northern Ontario, and we also share a studio/loft in downtown Toronto. It is now his office for writing and displaying his amazing collection of memorabilia and mine for painting. Happily, he is now cancer-free.

We have two amazing granddaughters, ages four and one, from my son Michael and daughter-in-law Carly. My daughter Meghan, and her husband Josh, have independent businesses as nutritionists, authors, and teachers. Meghan has an online culinary nutrition school, and Josh is a genius with his clients. He helped my husband get through his cancer, with a very positive outcome. Life is good. Grey is great!

GRAY8 TIPS & TECHNIQUES

To cleanse my hair I use an Organic Hydrating Shampoo by Onesta Hair Care Products. Occasionally I use L'Oreal Professionnel Serie Expert Silver Shampoo. I don't massage it in, and just let it sit for a few minutes before rinsing it out.

Pip Bacon
Age 45
Oxfordshire, England

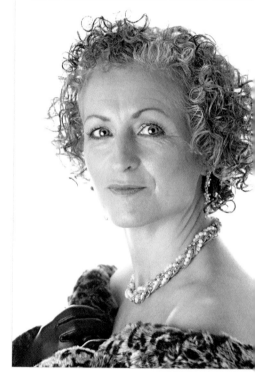

In the fall of 2002, I moved to a small village with thatched cottages, a school, church, a pub, a cricket pitch, and a village hall. It is so quintessentially English.

I have been very fortunate to have been blessed with three adorable (well, mostly!) boys, so our house is anything but quiet. Add in a Chocolate Labrador, and a Hungarian Vizsla, who think it's their duty, to bark at anything, and everything! So, as you can imagine, there is a degree of chaos that looms over our house on a daily basis.

I was born the third child of army parents, so my brothers and I moved around several times before we settled down near Liverpool. At eighteen, I moved to London to enroll in the Nightingale School of Nursing at St. Thomas Hospital, then sold my soul to the pharmaceutical industry, and began a career as a representative. Later, I took off to travel around the globe for nearly two years, working along the way to pay for my next adventure. Then, upon my return, I settled in Bristol for a few years before meeting my Darci (my future husband). Finally, we moved to an English Village in Middle England.

My love affair with hair colour started when I was about fifteen, bleaching my fringe with "Sun-In," a product that you sprayed on your hair, and used a blow-dryer to gradually lighten your hair. Obviously, it was designed for blondes and not brunettes, as my fringe ended up a lovely shade of ginger! I then moved to Henna (supposedly better for your hair as it is a natural product), but oh, the smell! My hair is very curly, (think spiral curls), so the ends would become very dry and grab the colour. I soon progressed to semi-permanent dye, since there were a variety of colours available. Then, in my late 20's,

I noticed the white random frizz popping through my mane of colour, so I moved to the hard stuff, the permanent dyes! That was it; I was hooked, and there was no going back now!

Slowly my colouring fix moved from once every eight weeks, to once a month. Then, in desperation, I added highlights to the top layers to try to avoid the halo of white, which frequented my hairline and saddened my heart. The problem is, as with all addictions, the product that made me feel better when I looked in the mirror, was gradually turning my hair crispy and frizzy, and costing me a fortune! Thoughts of ditching the dye, kept popping into my head more and more frequently, but the thought of being seen as "old and frumpy" kept me reaching for the bottle of dye.

Then, one summer day, I was up watching the cricket. There, I saw a young girl who had bleached her hair grey as a fashion statement! It looked great! It was right then, that I realised that being grey meant so much more than just the colour of your hair. For so many years, I had defined myself by my curly hair, never cutting it too short, because I was told that I shouldn't. Then I always coloured it, because I thought that I should and wanted to fit-in. But now I realise that those feelings of sadness (when I saw the white halo) were a result of the pressure that society puts on us if we don't colour. So, after much discussion with friends and family, I decided to take the plunge and go grey. I canceled my hair appointment, my hairdresser was not pleased with my decision; nor were several of my friends. One person actually asked, "How will you be able to keep your husband?" I started surfing the Internet and found lots of inspiration and have never looked back.

After about eight weeks of abstinence, I grew fidgety and quite obsessed by the shimmering colour starting to grow through. I was anxious to see if it aged me, and to see if my new colour would hold the curl. I lacked patience and hated the look of my badger stripe; it made me feel unkempt. And what colour was left in the curls, was brassy and crispy. Finally, I took the plunge and had it all chopped off into a short pixie, 1920's-style. The ends still held some colour, but I liked it. I looked slightly sophisticated with my new empowering style.

Then, in the summer of 2012, I received a call asking if I would be interested in being an extra in a new movie, but they wanted me to shave my head bald! Shiny bald! But guess what? I did it! I'm not so sure I would do it again, but it was so exciting being a part of something like that! After my head was shaved, I knew that in order to carry it off, I would need to wear a little more makeup and be very conscious of my dress choice. I was also very aware that there are a lot of people in the world who don't have any choice in being bald, and I did not want to offend anyone by falsely gaining pity after my stint in the movie was over. So I bought a wig and wore it for two weeks until I had a silver Marine buzz. Wearing the wig was fun! I got a long blonde style, and, with sunglasses I felt all "Hollywood!"

As my hair grew longer, not only did I love my new shimmers of silver, but the condition of my curls were noticeably bouncy and spirally again, just like when I was in my 20's. At fifteen months in, my hair has grown approximately eighteen centimetres, but due to its tight curl, I have a short bouncy bob with light white streaks at the front, blending into a darker salt and pepper at the back. Other than a rather large degree of serious long-hair envy, I have absolutely no regrets and cannot explain how liberating it felt to be free of the dye addiction that held me captive for so many years! My plan now is to grow my silver locks as long as I can, in the best possible condition I can. I am happy and in a great place in my life, and I hope to inspire other woman who dare to be grey! Follow your heart, and choose your own path!

GRAY8 TIPS & TECHNIQUES

I use Pro:Voke Touch of Silver Brightening Shampoo once a week. It helps brighten the colour and highlights the white. Recently, however, I have discovered products from White Hot Hair. My favorite is their awesome Shooshing Cream for silver locks, which adds style and helps maintain the shimmer.

Ros Johnstone
Age 49
Essex, UK

I have lived in the same town all my life, and love having family and friends nearby. I work part-time and am a mother of two, a fifteen year old daughter and a seventeen year old son. My son has severe autism and, unfortunately, has never spoken a word. My partner has two daughters, so needless to say, we spend a lot of time as a family, bowling, playing family games, eating out, watching movies, and everything else in between. We are always doing something!

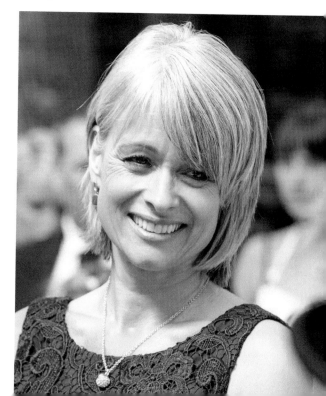

My first grey hairs started to appear when I was in my early 20's, so I decided to start colouring my hair then. I did it myself and used the same shade as my natural colour, so nobody really noticed. I continued doing it myself for a few years, but then I couldn't seem to get those grey hairs covered anymore, so I started going to the hairdresser.

Over the years, I would have my hairdresser change up the colour she was using on my hair. Sometimes I asked her to use a bit more red, or a shade darker, but I found that my hair was starting to get too dark, so I gradually had her lighten it. That way, I would be closer to my original colour. I always loved my natural hair colour the best, and was really beginning to miss it.

My hair grows very quickly, so I was going to the hairdresser's every four weeks, but after three weeks, I had a thin grey streak down the centre of my head and found it difficult to schedule my appointments around events I had coming up. I was slowly getting tired of all this.

In August 2013, I went to my regular hair colouring appointment, but this time, I was disappointed in how it turned out. When she was done, there were still grey strands showing up around my face! My grey hair was becoming resistant to the dye and had become more and more difficult to cover! I was upset because during this same time, I had a special event to attend. Since my son has severe autism, he has a carer whom I had nominated for a special award on ITV television. She was one of the three finalists, which meant, we were both going to appear on television and in the local newspaper. Overall she ended up coming in second place, which was fantastic as it was a huge competition!

On September 9, 2013, my carer and I were going to the Well Child Awards Ceremony, held at The Dorchester Hotel in London. Many celebrities attend this event, including Prince Harry and Rod Stewart. I had scheduled my hair appointment three days prior for this special occasion, but was disappointed again that the grey was not being covered.

After the event, I decided to go grey gracefully. I couldn't wait to start this journey. A friend of mine had transitioned, and I followed her story, never thinking that I would be joining her on this fantastic journey. I showed my partner her photos and asked what he thought. He said I would look fantastic with natural grey hair. I was fed up with colouring every three weeks. I had a photo taken for the local newspaper, and I hated the photo, I didn't like my hair colour, and I could see my roots peeking through. I got on the Internet and searched grey hair, and I liked what I saw, and, from that moment on, I decided this is what I'm going to do!

The last time I dyed my hair was in September 2013. I had long dark hair and was sure I wasn't going to cut it. As the grey started to come through, I felt so excited, because I really wanted this. During my transition, I had my hair highlighted three times to help with the demarcation line. I ended up with blonde hair, which I felt was a better contrast against the grey.

When I was nine months into my transition, I had my hair cut to shoulder-length; I loved this length and thought I would just keep getting it cut to this length until I was done. Then I started to get impatient, and I just wanted to get all my dyed hair cut off. I also had a wedding to attend, so I returned to my hair stylist and asked her to cut it short and layer it all up, and that was it. I was done at eleven months, and what a lovely feeling that was. I felt free and totally authentic; there is no one else who has my colour. I love being free of the dye!

GRAY8 TIPS & TECHNIQUES

In the beginning stages of my transition, I used Roux Fanci-Full Tween Time. You just paint it on your roots, and it washes out easily. It didn't cover the grey completely, but it helped to disguise my grey streak. My hair was dark, so at about three months in, (to make my skunk stripe less noticeable), I had my stylist put highlights throughout my hair, avoiding my grey roots.

I use ORS Olive Oil Creamy Aloe Shampoo and Conditioner and The Body Shop Coconut Oil Hair Shine, to smooth and define my hair. I love to finish with Pro:Voke Touch of Silver Hairspray.

My best advice would be to join an online grey support group where you can share ideas and gather tons of information!

Sandy Hicks
Age 53
Colorado

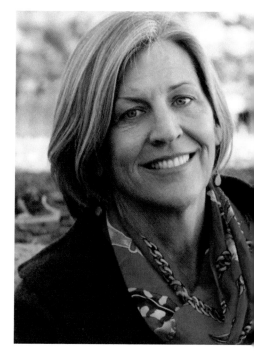

I'm not a conventional woman, by any means—I'm an engineer. I like math, and I am good at it! I have worked for almost 30 years in a predominately "male only" field, starting with road construction projects. I'm very athletic; I rowed for the University of Wisconsin Women's Crew team in the late 70's, when women didn't even have a locker room. Now they have a nicer locker room than the men! I bike and swim for exercise, and, most recently, I completed an open-water 10K swim, the length of Horsetooth Reservoir in Fort Collins, Colorado. I can also keep up with my husband and two sons ages (17), and (19), when it comes to skiing and bicycling.

My husband is going conventionally gray, but much slower than I am, (he only has gray on his temples). My mom went gray in her 60's, (after years of dyeing her hair). My nana, on the other hand, went gray in her mid-20's. She never dyed it, and loved it! She had a beautiful head of what she called silver hair, (you weren't allowed to call it gray)!

I think I finally came to the decision to stop dyeing my hair after my 100th visit to the salon, (or so it seemed). I was spending over three hours in the beautician's chair getting highlights and color. I mean, I liked her, but, I was spending more time with her than my own family. NO just kidding! But it really did seem like a waste of time, and, as costs went up, a waste of money. I mean, who was I kidding anyway? After a couple of weeks, the roots were pretty gray and didn't blend in well with the non-natural color. I don't think I had ever really thought that not dyeing was an option. I mean, everyone dyes their gray, right? (Okay, every WOMAN!)

My natural hair color growing up was brown, so I never really identified myself as a redhead, a blonde, or a raven-haired beauty. So, other than the fact that my hair was poker straight, the dyed hair colors I wore on my head throughout the years, were never my defining feature. When I was 48, I found a few clippings of silver-haired ladies in a magazine. Clutching them in my hand, I went into the hairdresser's and said, "Chop it off!" I left with a short pixie cut. I have had short hair a few times in the past 40 years, remember the wedge? So, getting my hair cut into a pixie wasn't that difficult of a decision to make. I figured it would be easier, and, being a busy working mom, it would be a big plus. And I was right! No dyeing! No sitting in the salon chair for hours on end! No chemical stews on my head! I loved it!

A couple things that shocked me and still shock me about being gray are:

1. Sometimes I don't recognize myself in pictures. I guess after years of being brownish-blonde I automatically assume, that's what I should look like!
2. People say the strangest things like, "If my gray hair was as pretty as yours, I'd let it grow out too." I mean, how do you know, if you never try it? Or they say "You can pull it off," like as if I'm wearing some weird or body-hugging fashion.

My father-in-law actually told me, "You wouldn't look so damn old if you'd just dye your hair." He's 83 and has a pure white head of hair and goatee. My cousin, (who is a year older than I am), recently said to me "I will never let myself go gray!" I believe, to each his own, I would never force my decision to go gray on anyone.

For women, dyeing our hair is really expected in our society. I think it's time we question this! Who says gray hair can't be beautiful? I find it interesting how people will be so careful with what they eat and drink, (eating only organic, etc.), but yet, they'll put toxic chemicals right on their skin (for hours each month), and never question it.

Now, I get almost as many compliments on my hair color as I do my haircut; a woman at the mall recently stopped me and told me that I looked stunning. I won't go back to dyeing. It was too much trouble, and actually I really like my gray hair! It is shiny and pretty and definitely a trademark of mine now!

GRAY8 TIPS & TECHNIQUES

I switch between Suave Shampoo and Pantene Shampoo, and condition with Aveda Dry Remedy Moisturizing Conditioner. For moisture and shine, I use Aveda Light Elements Smoothing Fluid, and I texturize with Garnier Fructis De-Constructed Pixie Play. I don't use a purple shampoo.

Once I transitioned to gray, I began to look at the colors in my wardrobe. I can't wear beige or off-white anymore, and I got rid of all my brown clothing.

My advice for anyone considering going gray, is be confident and ignore the nay-sayers. It is so worth it in the end!

Sara Davis Eisenman
Age 38
California

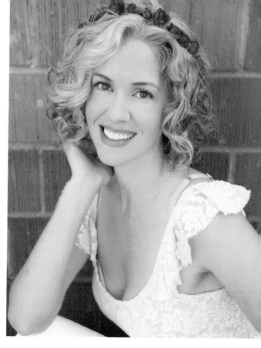

When I was 22, my hair went from its original black color to about 75 percent silver, almost overnight! This drastic change happened in response to a very traumatic time in my life. I remember feeling absolutely horrified, as I peered at my roots in the mirror; I associated the silver color much more with my mother, than myself. My mom had also gone gray early, and often had an unhappy relationship with her hair, lacking the money to color it regularly and feeling ashamed of her silver locks. Sometimes she simply wouldn't raise her head in public, despite the fact that she was and still is quite beautiful, inside and out.

I was determined not to suffer a similar fate, so I began coloring my hair every two to three weeks. My hair grows extremely fast, and coloring it was a never-ending task. I spent a great deal of time feeling ashamed, covering my head with hats and headbands to conceal either the ring of black dye left on my skin after coloring, or the annoying gray roots that became visible almost immediately after I got rid of the black ring! And so this continued, for about fifteen years, through college, graduate school, my professional life, a marriage, and two children. This secret I was always trying to keep hidden, was so much a part of my everyday existence, that the negative emotions I associated with it, became almost subliminal. There were times that I turned down invitations from friends because my roots were showing, or, like my mother, I simply could not raise my head or look others squarely in the eye because I was ashamed of my gray.

As I entered my 30's, I started to look around and notice that many others were harboring the same secret. It was no longer the case that I represented the anomaly, of a very young woman with gray hair. As I got older, I adapted to the norm. At that point, it suddenly occurred to me how strange it is that so many of us feel that we must color our hair in order to feel beautiful or accepted by society. It is one thing to choose to color, but it is another to feel less than, for choosing not to. I was starting to ask myself, "What is so wrong with my gray that I must continually cover it?" The layers of shame and unprocessed emotion associated with my hair began to surface, and, as I unpacked these layers, I was delighted to arrive at the following revelation: "There was nothing at all wrong with me, or my gray hair!"

I began to see my shiny silver roots as pretty, not ugly or shameful at all. The next trick was to try and figure out how I was going to get through the transition. I approached several hairdressers with the idea of growing out my gray hair, and, to my surprise, they tried to dissuade me, and a couple of them flat-out refused to help. After my second child's birth (when I was 36), the abstract notion of growing out my gray roots, soon became a reality, as I was so busy caring for my toddler and newborn, that visiting the hairdresser was simply not an option. At this time, coloring my hair myself was about the last thing on planet Earth I cared about, as I fell into bed thoroughly worn-out each night.

I realized that this was my chance to go for it. I was already well into the awkward stage, and there was no point, not to mention no time, to color it again. Most importantly, I wanted to be a champion for other women and to validate their authentic beauty by confidently representing my own, and, that desire to empower others drove my decision more than anything else.

My transition was not without its challenges. The first few months, in particular, were difficult as my hair was about as two-toned as it gets. At this time, I returned to my favorite hairdresser, who is also a dear friend, (even though it meant traveling farther from my home). She was very supportive and helped my transition enormously by removing much of my former black color and giving me a stylish shorter cut to speed up the process.

Throughout the process, I chose to simply be okay with each and every stage, to place my focus on my beautiful family and the many blessings in my life, to surround myself with loving people, and to keep breathing. Perhaps most importantly, I chose to look in the mirror and say to myself, "You are beautiful," even when society's interpretation of my reflection was most likely the contrary.

The outcome of my year-long transition is a deep, true self-love and sense of confidence that I have never experienced before. I stopped looking at myself and all my flaws with harsh judgment, (which I wasn't fully consciously aware of doing in the first place), and instead, I began to look at myself with a softer, more accepting gaze. This new self-acceptance applied not only to my hair, but also to the sum total of myself. I realized that holding myself to the standard of society's version of beauty (or the way I interpreted that standard), had been holding me back from developing and stepping-out in other areas of my life: my intellect, my compassion, and my wisdom. Freeing my gray hair was an important key to freeing myself, and it's a decision I'm so very grateful to have made.

It has now been eighteen months since my transition to silver began, and the gifts of growing out my natural hair continue to reveal themselves. Though I had no idea how this big change in my life would be received by others, I am now approached by people everywhere I go, who tell me how much they like my hair. Many confide that I have inspired them to grow out their own natural color, and this ability to inspire others gives me a feeling like no other. My transition to silver also gave me a forum on which to publicly share my love of natural beauty, which also taps very powerfully and seamlessly into my work as an energy healer and nutrition counselor. The process of eliminating chemicals from my life in favor of natural, earth-based practices has made its way into every area of my life, from beauty and hygiene products to household cleaners, greatly improving my health and quality of life. I could not have predicted all these wonderful changes, nor would I have tried to—I simply knew that I had to follow my heart, and I am incredibly glad I did. I hope my story will also inspire other women to see and embrace their unique, one-of-a-kind beauty, for beauty truly does come from within.

I am a mother, energy healer, nutrition counselor, writer, and public figure. I graduated with high honors from UC Berkeley with a Bachelor's degree in Neuroscience and Philosophy, and also hold a

Master's degree in Culture and Performance from UCLA. As a product of a difficult childhood in which both my parents were diagnosed as mentally ill and disabled, I fulfill the archetype of the wounded healer. In my work, I specialize in helping others heal from trauma and deepen their mind and body connection in order to transform their health and lives for the better.

GRAY8 TIPS & TECHNIQUES

My hair care regime is simple. I use sulfate-free products and wash my hair with DermOrganic Argan Oil Shampoo and Conditioner. I style my hair with Argan oil or coconut oil, and let my hair air-dry naturally. When my hair occasionally begins to acquire yellow tones, I shampoo with baking soda and rinse with vinegar and water.

My overall beauty philosophy is to use as few chemicals as possible, and to intervene only minimally, with what nature has given me. I truly believe in beauty from the inside out, so my primary beauty products are a good, organic diet high in nutrients and nourishing fats, mindfulness practices such as meditation and yoga, detoxifying baths, and, of course, plenty of laughter and love.

Photo credit: Jennifer Quest

Sharon Rogers
Age 50
Colchester, UK

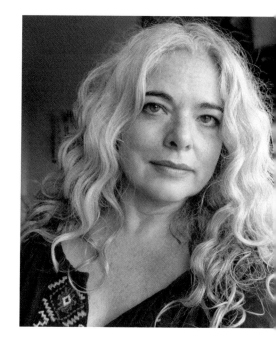

I was fifteen years old when I spotted my first grey hair. I was upstairs in my bedroom, saw the silvery strand, and let out a scream. My mother, who was downstairs, assumed I'd seen a spider. At the time, she didn't have any grey hair, so having her daughter find one was surprising to both of us. My father had been greying since his teens, so I really shouldn't have been surprised at all.

As a teenager, I loved experimenting with my hair and dyed it every colour imaginable. Often, it would be three different colours in the space of a week, though mostly I alternated between a pre-raphaelite red and a very dark brown, the colour I was born with.

I was in my mid 20's when I became aware that my roots were growing out. There was a lot of white in there! It didn't worry me, because I was still changing my hair colour every other week, (not to cover grey), but because, I enjoyed using the different colours, and changing my appearance regularly. This continued into my 30's, and it was towards the end of that decade, that I began to see the emerging grey as a problem. Growing out the dye, did not even occur to me back then, and covering the roots began to feel like a chore.

It was in the summer of 2007, just before my 44th birthday, that I began to entertain the idea of growing out the dye to see my natural hair colour. I mentioned the idea to my mother, who was quite frankly horrified (she is now in her 70's and still dyeing her hair). I bought a book on going grey, and was fascinated by the stories of women who had gone natural. I was tempted to try it, but it seemed like such a daunting idea. My hair was very long at the time and dyed a dark brown. The roots would be very noticeable. So I put the book away and continued dyeing my hair until the end of that year.

January always feels like a time for new beginnings, and, at the beginning of 2008, when my roots started to appear, I thought about not covering them. I mentioned it to my mother again, and she was still horrified at the idea, and told me "I'd look old," and that it would be a mess growing it out. I thought she could be right, but somehow I didn't care about all that. I was curious to see what was actually under there, after 30 years of dyeing. So, I announced it to everyone what I was planning to do. A couple of months before my last dye, I had gone quite a lot shorter in hair length, which made the idea less daunting. I watched my roots coming in and was eager to get rid of the dye as quickly as possible, having three haircuts over the next few weeks. By the beginning of March, I was ready to be completely natural and told the hairdresser to cut off ALL the dye, no matter how short the results.

I liked the silver; I liked how soft and healthy my natural hair felt after years of being damaged by chemicals. I felt liberated and I loved it. I wanted to have long hair again and went through a year of feeling incredibly frumpy, as my hair went through the stages of growing out from the short cut. This was difficult. Sometimes I would look in the mirror and see my grandmother looking back at me. I had no urge to dye my hair again; I just wanted to have it long.

Eventually, two-and-a-half years later, my hair was a reasonable length again and I was happy. Then, something strange happened. I began to think I looked old and drab. I missed the days when I would change my hair colour every other week. I wasn't happy. I saw myself in some photographs and thought I looked old and boring, and I didn't like it. So, I made a decision, and, within a few short hours, I was slathering my hair in bright red dye. I liked the results, for a couple of days... anyway. Then I hated how fake it began to look, and decided to tone it down and go brown again. Soon the roots started coming in, and, before I knew it, I was back on the treadmill, having to cover my roots every two to three weeks. I soon regretted what I'd done, but could not face going short again, especially after all that time I spent, growing my hair back out. I bought a box of hair dye remover, which lightened it a little. I then bleached my hair several times in the hopes that somehow I could get out the dye and have my natural hair back. But all that did was ruin my hair and the resultant yellow tones made me look ill. I decided to go very dark again, almost black this time, and put up with the tyranny of the roots for the next couple of years.

The decision to transition for the second time happened in the summer of 2012. I was on holiday in Italy, and I knew full well that my roots would need tending to while I was away, so I took a box of dye with me. Towards the end of the holiday, I was in my room dyeing my hair instead of enjoying myself at the pool. I thought how ridiculous this was, and remembered how free I'd felt when I didn't have to think about my roots. A couple of days later, I visited an old Italian hill town. In the evenings, the men and women would sit outside their homes, and, as I was watching them, something really struck me. Most of these women had very harshly dyed hair, very flat, and black looking. They were mature women, and the stark black hair did them no favours. It certainly didn't make them look young. There was one Italian woman, though, the landlady of the place we were staying at, who had long, natural hair, streaked with grey. I thought how beautiful and natural she looked, compared with the other women.

When I came home, I looked at the photographs of myself in Italy. My hair was black as coal and not very flattering. It was then and there that I decided I had to transition again. I decided that I would go very short again, knowing that for me, once the decision was made, I would want the dye out as quickly as possible. I had made five visits to the hairdresser's in quick succession, and, within four months, I was done. My hair was VERY SHORT again, but free of the dye. That was fifteen months ago, and I've been growing out the short cut ever since. I have not regretted it even once. I am aware that, (like last time), I may sometimes feel I look drab, but this time I know it has nothing to do with my natural hair. On the days I look drab; it's usually because I'm wearing an item of clothing that doesn't flatter me, or in a colour that no longer looks good against my skin tone. If I had realised that the first time round, I never would have returned to the dye. This time, I have no doubts; I am very sure that I will never dye my hair again.

GRAY8 TIPS & TECHNIQUES

I have a very basic hair care routine. I wash my hair every day with an inexpensive shampoo and conditioner and occasionally use Pantene Pro-V Silver Expressions Shampoo, or mix a little baking soda into the shampoo, then follow with a white vinegar/water rinse to brighten my hair. After conditioning, I use the plopping technique mentioned in "Curly Girl The Handbook" by Lorraine Massey with Michele Bender. Once my hair has stopped dripping, I scrunch in a little John Frieda Frizz Ease Serum, and allow my hair to air-dry naturally. That's it! The less I fiddle with my hair, the better it looks!

Remember that after transitioning, it may take some time for you to adjust to your new colouring. Experiment with clothing and makeup colours, as you may need to make some changes to better complement your natural hair.

Shelby Zehner

Age 56

Pennsylvania

I actually started coloring my hair when I was fifteen. Going blonde seemed to be the thing to do, when all you had was mousey brown hair. Coloring my hair made me feel pretty. I kept up with the blonde until 1977, when I gave birth to a red-haired baby boy, whose hair was always the topic of conversation. So, I decided to give red a try myself. I liked the red color, so, for the next several years, I alternated between red and blonde. I colored according to whatever mood I was in at the time, but my old standby color was blonde.

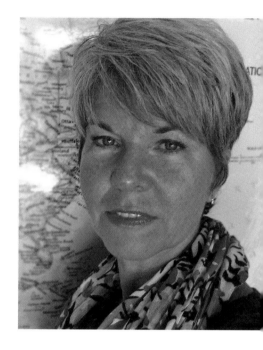

I was a redhead back in the 80's when my marriage broke up. My boss at the time, (later to become my husband,) mentioned at one point, that he was not a fan of red hair. I kept it red for a little while longer, but then went back to dyeing it blonde again.

At this point in my life, I quit coloring my own hair and started going to the salon. It was fun being pampered and fussed over. I got highlights and lowlights and was in the chair for hours. I never minded. It was ME time, and I loved all the girls in the salon.

Fast forward to 2013, and I now have five children that are (38), (36), (32), (15), and (13). I have nine grandchildren and one on the way. I spend every summer, (June through August), in Key West. The last few summers were hard on my hair, as I had no desire to seek out a professional hairdresser in Key West. All summer I would walk around with a "lit-up runway" on the top of my head. By the end of the summer my bleached-blonde hair, became so parched and brittle-looking from the harsh sun. Getting home and getting my hair toned down was always in the forefront of my mind. That's when I began thinking about going gray.

So, this past July, while in Key West, I texted my hairdresser and told her my plan of going gray. When I returned home, she toned down my color, added a few lowlights here and there (leaving my roots alone), and trimmed my hair. I told my four girls my plan. To my surprise, everyone thought it was a cool idea. Even my teen age daughters were on board. My husband, on the other hand, was NOT! My husband doesn't like short hair, and was open with his negative feelings, when I went the pixie route. But, me being me, I just forged ahead, thinking that when I had beautiful sparkly gray hair, he would come around.

Early December 2013, was my last trim appointment. Now I am color-free. My hair is still shorter than I would like it to be, but it feels wonderful! So soft! My colored hair was so dry feeling, that this is a nice change for me. I would love to grow it to shoulder-length. That would give me multiple styling options.

While in Key West over the Christmas holiday, a man who takes care of our property (while we are not there), called me over to chat. This was the first time he saw my gray hair. He told me, that as my gay friend, he thought I should hear from him, that my gray hair made me look ten years older; and that he had been talking about it with my husband, who also felt the same way! This comment was pretty upsetting, mostly because my own husband had been discussing my hair with that man, and not sticking up for my side! I think he should have had my back, no matter what he thought in private!

I was a dental assistant for about fifteen years. After the birth of my two youngest daughters, I have become a full-time stay-at-home mom. Along with driving the girls to their various activities, I enjoy baking, reading, walking, and running. I have participated in several 5K's and Half Marathons. Staying in shape and healthy is important to me, especially after having two kids later in life. I want to be around as long as I can for them.

I am hoping that my hubby's dislike for my hair will come to an end when this short hair grows to a more feminine length. He has never been a fan of short hair on me. I think that going gray and going short was just too much for him all at once. But—it is my hair, and I do what makes me feel pretty. However, I do hope he will come around, because I will never color my hair again.

GRAY8 TIPS & TECHNIQUES

I use AG Hair Cosmetics Sterling Silver Shampoo and Conditioner to keep my hair beautiful. I also use CHI Silk Infusion Reconstructing Complex to keep my hair shiny. At this point, with my hair being so short, I just wash and air-dry it. Sometimes I use a curling-iron to just bend bits and pieces so I don't look like I'm wearing a helmet.

My makeup has also changed. Instead of peachy cheeks, I've changed to more of a berry shade for cheeks and lips. I think the hair color also brings out my blue eyes!

My wardrobe used to include a lot of neutral colors, but now includes more jewel-tones. I think these bright colors make my hair look more silvery, which I love!

Suzanne Henderson

Age 53
Michigan

I've had a few gray hair strands since I was sixteen, but did not start dyeing my hair until my early 20's. I began dyeing my hair, not to cover the gray, but because I wanted to try out the different hair colors. But, as time went on, I began to color less. Then, in 1993 (after having my first born), the gray began to cover more than just my temples. I did not realize the power of gray hair! I started out dyeing my hair midnight black, but the silver strands did not cover in the same way as the rest of my hair. Under office lighting, it looked like I had a purple halo at my root line. It was a purple mess! My next dye job was then jet black. I continued to dye my hair black, until I found myself needing a root touch-up every two-and-a-half to three weeks.

Then one day, I encountered a beautiful lady who was rocking a short, all-white pixie. Thinking my hair could look like hers, I decided that I would grow my hair out. I stopped dyeing my hair around early 2011. My decision to stop dyeing my hair came pretty easily. I stood in front of the mirror, parted my hair in the center, and found that my gray roots far outnumbered my black roots! My gray hair ratio was about 90 percent!

During my going gray process, I began to utilize some home-whitening remedies, but my hair started to break off. My cute skunk bob

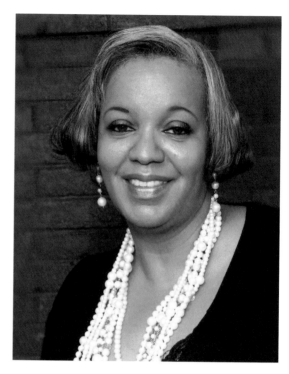

was now patchy and damaged, so I went to a stylist and had all the black ends cut off. It was an immediate transformation. This cut fully transitioned me to gray. But I still did not understand the sensitivity of certain products, or sun on gray hair. In the summer of 2012, my hair seemed to turn yellow. Later, I realized that the combination of heat and styling products was causing a dark, singed look. Rather than just letting Mother Nature take its course, I tried a number of products to whiten my hair. I used baking soda, apple cider vinegar, volume peroxide, and a mix of products, but they only damaged my hair even further. It was then that I decided to visit the same salon, of the woman who was rocking the all-white pixie. But because my hair was damaged, I had to get a shorter pixie cut. The stylist informed me that my shade of color was not white, but more silver. At first, I was disappointed, but, once my hair began to grow out, I started receiving loving compliments, and I embraced my silver hair.

In pictures where all my friends have dark hair, I stand out. My friends have started calling me the "Silver Fox." Currently, I maintain a short ear-length cut, allowing me to curl my hair tightly, or wear it straight. I receive more compliments on my silver hair today (from both sexes); than I ever did the whole time my hair was black!

My career over the last fifteen years has been in Human Resources; I am a natural peace maker. I would like to be more involved with encouraging, and mentoring women seeking employment. I am a single mother of one son, and my hobby is resale-shopping and stocking for Outta My Closet on Shopify. My dream is to own and operate a mobile consignment venue someday. My going silver has also inspired my mom; she loved my silver hair and decided to transition as well. She stopped dyeing her hair on Mother's Day of 2013.

GRAY8 TIPS & TECHNIQUES

My favorite hair products include: Clairol Shimmer Lights Shampoo and Conditioner and SoftSheen Carson Bantu Yellow-Out Conditioner. For shine, I use Proclaim Moisturizing Oil Sheen Spray and Cantu Shea Butter. I shampoo and blow-dry my hair at least once a week and use a flatiron to straighten it.

I like to wear colors that allow my silver to stand out more. I usually don't wear a lot of browns and yellows, and I tend to gravitate towards bold colors, as well as the staples of black, white, and silver.

With silver hair, I have made a few makeup changes. I utilize paler, softer tones, as opposed to the darker liners and lipsticks.

I often hear women say, "If my hair would be silver like yours, I would do it in a heartbeat." My advice to anyone wanting to transition would be; you will never know unless you give it a try! Plus you can always change it back if you don't like it! Just go for it! Confidence is the key!

Viv McRoy
Age 58
Lake District UK

Although I am 58, I am probably about 27 in my head. I live in a beautiful part of the UK, have three brilliant kids, (two girls and a boy), and two of the most amazing grandchildren.

One of my favourite past-times is reading. I belong to a book club, but really, we drink wine and gossip, but book club sounds better! I absolutely love music, especially Tamla Motown and Northern Soul Music and still love to dance. I enjoy going to live music concerts and am lucky to be just an hour away from both Liverpool and Manchester, where we often go to see live bands. I also enjoy the theatre and the cinema.

My son and his family live in Liverpool, and my husband Dave and I love going to visit and

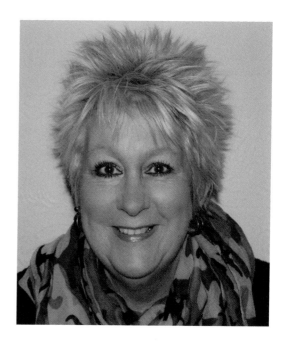

babysit, while soaking up the history and culture of the most amazing city in England. I work with kids (from ages eight to eighteen) with emotional, behavioral, and educational difficulties, who, believe me, are my harshest critics! Those kids are not for the easily offended! I love my job with a passion; although it is very challenging, it is also very rewarding. The kids love my hair, but are convinced that it's dyed this colour!

I started colouring my hair for fun, when I was fourteen-years-old. Then in my mid-20's, I started noticing a few grey hairs scattered throughout. My dad's side of the family all started going grey prematurely, so it came as no surprise. I continued colouring my hair for the next 31 years, using highlights, lowlights, and every colour you can possibly imagine. To be honest, the grey thing just sort of crept up on me, the older I got, the greyer I got, and I found myself colouring more frequently.

Once I was in my mid-40's, I decided to stop colouring all together. I just left the silver alone to see what would happen, and found myself rapidly going grey. I wasn't too bothered by it, and actually, I really liked my new grey colour! I found it easy to transition and never faltered once. I kept my hair very short, and it took me all of four months, if that, to fully transition.

Now that I'm completely silver, I find it slightly hilarious, that for many years, I went to the hairdresser's and "paid" for silver highlights, while now I have my own free silver highlights! Vidal Sassoon was a favourite place to go in the 70's. I must have spent a small fortune colouring my hair over the years! I probably could have bought a small house! LOL!

The number of positive comments I get never ceases to amaze me! I can honestly say it was not a big deal for me to go grey! I love my silver hair and can't ever imagine colouring it again! I think in the UK, lots of women go grey, and it's just not an issue. People say I'm brave, but I'm not sure why? I am very lucky with the colour I have, and everyone thinks I dyed it like this! Can't win! We travel to Marrakech quite often, and my hair is a constant source of amusement to the Moroccans, who don't seem to go grey! But I certainly am GREY AND PROUD!

GRAY8 TIPS & TECHNIQUES

My youngest daughter is a hairdresser, so she devised the cut I wear now. I have had it for a good while because it's so easy to take care of, and I get lots of compliments! I use L'Oreal Series Expert Silver Shampoo once a week to keep my hair at its best, it's a wonderful product! I never use conditioner, as I find it makes my hair very limp. I am a huge fan of DaxWax, the cheapest thing ever, so I wash, blast, and wax!

I love wearing makeup, especially bold lipstick. I also have a large selection of funky earrings, which go great with my short hair. Bright scarves are a big favourite of mine; the brighter, the better!

gray8
skincare
& makeup

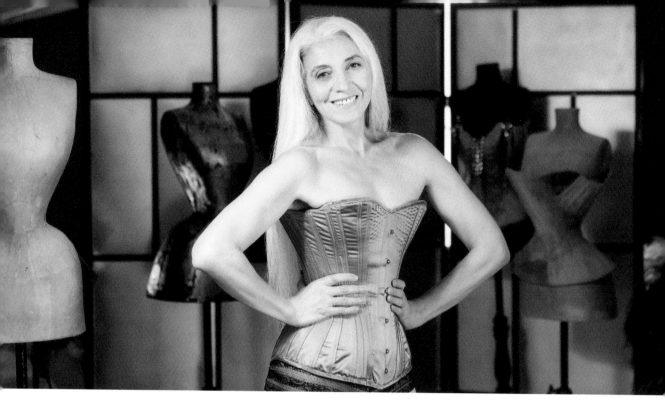

the skinny on skincare

SUNCARE

As a Licensed Esthetician, it is a privilege to be able to educate people on the importance of skincare, and help them to achieve their best skin. The sun will have the largest influence on how your skin will age. If you are ignoring your skin, and not using the proper sunscreen, it will definitely have a direct impact on your skins overall health. The sunlight that reaches us has two types of harmful rays, UVA and UVB. Over exposure to either can damage the skin. UVA (Ultraviolet Aging), are long rays that penetrate deep into the dermis (the skin's thickest layer). Over exposure can lead to hyperpigmentation (brown spots), premature aging, and skin cancer. UVB (Ultraviolet Burning), are short waves that will usually burn the superficial layers of the skin and can cause permanent skin cell damage. UVB rays are the same rays that tan your skin. The intensity of UVB rays will vary, depending on the time of day, season, and your geographic location. Use a sunscreen daily with SPF (Sun Protection Factor) 30-50 and re-apply it according to directions. Also don't forget your sunglasses to protect the skin around the eye area. It is never too late to start taking good care of your skin!

SKINCARE BASICS

Nutrition, health, lifestyle, stress, and environment/pollutants influence skin health, and can speed up the aging process. I can always recognize a smokers' skin, by the skins yellowish/gray appearance. Skincare starts with nutrition and water intake. You have heard the saying, "You are what you eat." Well—it's true! What you put in your body will have a direct effect on the aging of the skin. Poor nutrition, tobacco, drugs, and alcohol, all have a direct impact, on skin and overall health. To keep everything in good working order, practice good skincare from the inside out!

Some people just have good genes, darn it! But if you take good care of your skin (the largest organ of the body), it will definitely reward you back! There are many antioxidants on the market that you can take to help improve your skin's overall health. These antioxidants are included in many products. There are only a few prescriptions on the market that can actually help reduce already-damaged skin, i.e.; retinol and prescription-strength retinoid, such as Retin-A etc. Prescription creams are expensive, so for most of us—it comes down to good basic skincare.

CLEANSE - EXFOLIATE - MOISTURIZE & PROTECT

Proper cleansing techniques, along with moisturizing dehydrated skin, are imperative for healthy skin. Even if you don't wear makeup it's important to cleanse your face daily to remove air-borne pollutants. Basic skincare includes:

1. Cleanse: 2 remove makeup/pollutants
2. Exfoliate: 2 remove impurities/dead skin cells
3. Moisturize: 2 nourish
4. Sunscreen: 2 protect

You should cleanse your face twice daily: In the morning when you get up, and at night before you go to bed. Remove mascara with gentle eye makeup remover, or makeup remover towelettes. Avoid pulling and tugging around the delicate eye area. Remove excess makeup with a makeup remover towelette, and follow-up with a gentle non-drying facial cleanser. Lather cleanser between hands and apply to face and neck. To cleanse neck, use top side of both hands, fingers only, (slightly bent), using straight-upward strokes (effleurage); alternate hands in quick secession. To cleanse face, use a circular motion, you can use your hands, or a purifying sonic brush. Rinse thoroughly with lukewarm water and gently pat skin dry with a soft cloth. Many Licensed Estheticians' use

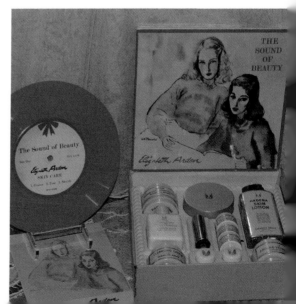

soft cloth diapers on their clients' and have found them to be very gentle on the skin. To exfoliate, use a clarifying lotion/toner (avoid eye area and lips). A clarifying lotion/toner not only removes remaining residue/impurities and dead skin cells, but also prepares the skin so that the moisturizer can penetrate the skin and do its job! There are many clarifiers on the market; Dickinson's Original Witch Hazel Pore Perfecting Toner is very affordable; 100 percent all-natural ingredients and fragrance-free. Moisturize according to your skin type and finish your routine by applying a sunscreen. Once a week, treat yourself to a mask or gentle facial scrub to refine and smooth the skin. Bottom line—proper cleansing affects the overall health and appearance of your skin!

SKIN TYPE

In order to take proper care of your skin and purchase the correct facial products, you will need to know your skin type. There are six basic skin types:

1. Dry
2. Very Dry
3. Normal
4. Oily
5. Combination
6. Sensitive

An example of combination skin is: (N/D), normal to dry and (N/O), normal to oily. Combination skin occurs when the T-Zone (nose, forehead, and chin) are one skin type, and the cheeks are another. Many people have combination skin. You can get your skin typed by a Dermatologist, Esthetician, Cosmetic Beauty Advisor/Consultant, or online by answering a few simple questions. Your skin type can change throughout the seasons and years, so it's important to get re-typed and stay current with your product applications.

EYE CARE

The thinnest skin on the body is the eyelids, so it is important to treat the eye area gently. Always use your ring finger when applying eye products, to avoid tugging and pulling the delicate skin. Using an eye cream, will give you just the right amount of moisture you need. Too heavy of a moisturizer will give you bags and sags. When applying your face cream, do not get to close to the eye area to avoid white bumps under the eye area, or puffiness etc. The skin underneath the eye area is much thinner and needs a moisturizing cream designed specifically for that area. I recommend Clinique, All About Eyes Rich; it diminishes circles and puffiness and softens fine lines. At 62, I have witnessed firsthand the benefits of using an eyecream. There are several different formulations to choose from, depending upon your specific needs. If I had to choose just one skincare product, eye cream would win hands-down.

BEAUTY SLEEP & SKIN

When you sleep, your body goes into overdrive to heal itself, so nighttime is the perfect time to pull out all the stops and do your part! If you have problematic skin, dig out your facial prescription. If your arms and legs are dry, grab the body lotion. Then open your nighttime beauty bag and pull out your eye cream, lip balm, and your best face cream to treat, soften, and moisturize your skin, Lie back on your satin pillowcase with your pineapple up-do, clear your head of all the drama, and get some shut-eye; about eight hours should do the trick. Then you will awaken to your most beautiful graylicious self!

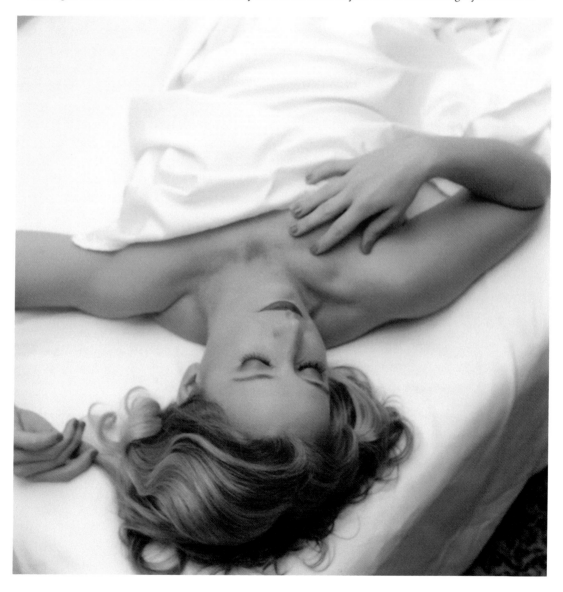

eyebrows 101

The perfect eyebrow can be measured using three lines. We have all seen the diagrams showing how our eyebrows should look. Even so, I still shake my head every time I work on my own brows and wonder whatever happened to them! But, as an Esthetician, I know first-hand that I am hardly alone. I have yet to come across the perfect brow, at least not without a little help from a few friends like; tweezers, wax, pencils, powders, etc. So, on that note—get your eyebrow pencil out, and let's start measuring!

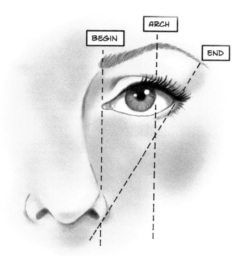

The eyebrow starts with a vertical line, measuring from the outer edge of the nose (straight up) to the inner corner of the eye and up.

The eyebrow arch (high point of brow) is measured with a vertical line, measuring from the outer circle/edge of the eyes iris, straight upward.

The eyebrow ends with an angle line, measuring from the outer corner of the nostril to the outer corner of the eye.

It's important to remember that this is only a guideline. Not everyone will have perfectly shaped brows. Work with your own natural brows to enhance what you already have. Everyone's eyebrows are unique to that particular individual. If everyone walked around with the exact same brows, it would look pretty funny, don't you think? Do not let trends dictate how you shape your eyebrows! Remember that eyebrows help frame your face, and define your look!

We love gray hair, but gray eyebrows? Not so much!

WHAT HAPPENED TO MY BEAUTIFUL BROWS?

As we age, our eyebrows become thinner, and if that's not bad enough, the ones that do come in seem to be growing in different directions! You may start to notice a few gray hairs, along with some crazy thick hairs as well. But you really need to give it some thought before you tweeze those little guys out. A hair may not come back to replace it, and you might be left with a bare spot instead! (The baby boomers know exactly what I'm talking about!) Remember: use brow scissors to trim, color to fill-in the gaps, and brow wax to hold.

Brows should complement your face not distract from it!

WHAT COLOR SHOULD MY EYEBROWS BE?

That is the multi-million-dollar question! If you do a search on the Internet, you will literally find every answer under the sun. It seems that every makeup artist has a different opinion, so who is right? The old "rule of thumb" is a shade or two darker than your natural hair color. But it is obvious that the person who made up this rule did not take into account that anyone would ever let their hair go gray. A shade or two darker than white hair may not cut it, and that is where many get lost. If you have a mixture of gray shades in your hair, and your eyebrows are naturally dark, my bet is they already match one of the shades you are sporting, and that everything blends together perfectly. If you have black eyebrows with all-white hair, do not use a black brow pencil; use a shade or two lighter to soften your brows. A good way to make sure you are using the right color is simply look in the mirror! You should see your entire face. If all you see are eyebrows; then you have answered your own question.

Don't let your eyebrows enter a room before you do! Banish bushy brows!

EYEBROW COLORS FOR GRAY HAIR

Here are a few eyebrow shades that work gray8 with gray hair: blonde, taupe, gray, charcoal, and certain shades of brown. If you cannot find an eyebrow shade that works for you, consider using an "eye pencil" or "eye shadow" instead (there are plenty of shades to choose from). Some women have brown

eyes, brown in their eyebrows, and brown in their natural hair, so they can carry off a brown shade easily. There are many different shades of brown, so if you are using a brown; avoid red and yellow undertones. Always remember, your eyebrow color may look gray8 in the bathroom mirror, but may appear unnatural in outdoor lighting.

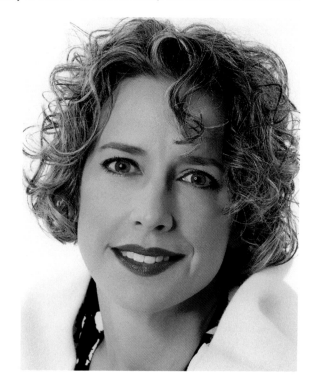

Eyebrows help frame your face! Wear color on your brows!

EYEBROW FAVORITES

If you have dark eyes and dark in your hair, check-out Chanel Crayon Sourcils Eyebrow Pencil Brun (40). It's the perfect choice for a "brown" eyebrow pencil. Chanel also makes a Blond Clair (10) eyebrow pencil that looks gray8 with gray hair. Unfortunately it was not the right shade for me, so I ended up giving it to my daughter Cheyenne. It was the perfect shade for her fair skin and blue eyes, and complemented her dye-free hair. If you want a darker shade of gray, Clinique makes a Charcoal Brow Shaper. Apply it with a light hand and use your spooly brush to blend. If you need to add color to your already existing brows, Lancôme has a brow groomer called Modèle Sourcils (color taupe) and of course, there is always Lancôme's "tried and true" taupe pencil. Another good choice is Bonne Bell: Eye Definer Pencil Pebble (34001). You can soften any color by using a spooly brush and blending to the desired shade. Then once you have everything figured out, your natural eyebrows may change; causing you to search for a new shade! UGH!

Fuller brows look more youthful than pencil thin brows!

EYEBROW COLOR APPLICATION

There are eyebrow dyes, gels, colored waxes, pencils, mascara's, and powders you can use to color and fill-in your eyebrows. Before you start, a helpful tip is to always brush your eyebrows first. Brushing them will remove any dead skin cells and create smoothness. You may get a little pink skin from the stimulation, but it will soon disappear. Also the stimulation is good for the brows and may encourage growth. You can easily shape your brows by using an eyebrow pencil or small angled brush. If you have sparse, patchy, or thin brows, fill them in with a pencil, using short, feathery strokes. Once you have your eyebrows shaped, apply powder color (using a sponge applicator). If you have full brows you may prefer eyebrow mascara instead. To keep eyebrows perfectly in place, use transparent eyebrow gel or wax to hold.

A well-groomed and nicely colored brow will not draw attention to itself!

TWEEZING OR PLUCKING?

When I was attending Esthetic's school, I once used the term PLUCK instead of TWEEZE. As soon as the teacher heard me she immediately (at the top of her lungs) corrected me, in front of the class. "You pluck a chicken; you tweeze an eyebrow!" The scary part was, (believe it or not), I could actually relate to what she was saying! As a child, I actually helped my mom pluck a chicken. I mean, what are the odds in that? LOL! Now everytime I hear or see the word PLUCK, I think of that dang chicken! Needless to say, I did not make that mistake again. Pluck, pluck, pluck, pluck, pluck!

4 TIPS 4 SHAPING YOUR EYEBROWS

1. First and foremost, let your eyebrows grow out.
2. Have a Licensed Esthetician set the blueprint for your eyebrow shape.
3. Trim before you tweeze. Comb brows up and trim "one hair at a time."
4. Use slanted Tweezerman Tweezers.

Both eyebrows should match in size, color, and shape!

OVER-TWEEZING EYEBROWS

If you are tweezing your eyebrows every day, or every couple of days, it's time to put the tweezers away, preferably under lock and key if possible. Only dig them out every couple of weeks, at the most! If you must get them out, tweeze that hair on your chin or upper lip instead. Give your eyebrows a chance to grow out and take shape on their own, before you start tweezing them. Do not tweeze your eyebrows while using a magnifying mirror. I have a 20 magnifying mirror, so, unless my friends are all walking around with a 20 magnifier lens attached to their glasses, they are not going to see those little hairs, anyway!

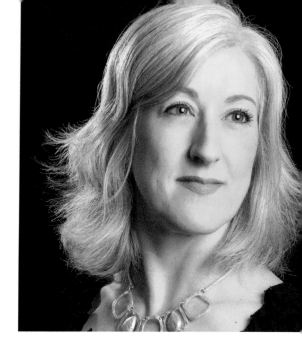

Back in the 70's, when I was in high school, tweezing your eyebrows was in style. Some girls even carried their tweezers in their pockets, just in case a stray hair would miraculously appear. But no one ever told us about over-tweezing, and that our eyebrow hairs may not grow back! For some, they did, but for others; not so much. If you make a mistake while tweezing, STOP and STEP BACK! Do not make the same mistake with the other brow. Instead, fill in the "mistake brow" with a pencil or powder until it grows back out.

Eyebrows don't take up a lot of space-on-your-face, so don't give them less space by over-tweezing!

WHAT IF YOU DON'T HAVE EYEBROWS?

If you have a small number of eyebrow hairs (even just a few fuzzy ones), tinting them with eyebrow dye (along with the skin underneath), will give you more of a brow. But the dye will fade, so you will need to do it again, (brow dye is less harsh than hair dye). If you have zero hairs, you can create eyebrows by using a pencil and a stencil. Or last but not least you can also use eyebrow wigs.

Don't tweeze those little white hairs out, hold onto them for "safe keeping!" You may need them later!

WHAT ABOUT BROW TATTOO'S?

Brow tattoos can look harsh, unnatural, and outdated if not done correctly. Also, a "mistake on your face" will stare you down in the mirror every day. You do not want someone to draw a single line across your brow bone and call that an eyebrow. They need to use several tiny, hair-like strokes. Remember, brow tattoos are permanent, so they will be staring back at you for a very long time!

Don't let a bad tattoo, stare you in the face!

gray8 makeup apps

Enhancing your appearance with the use of cosmetics (kosmetikos); dates all the way back to the ancient Egyptians. Kohl, lead, cinnabar, red iron oxide, and soot (from lamps), were just a few of the ingredients used in ancient makeup preparations. There have been numerous lotions, potions, toiletries, and, beauty gadgets made throughout the years, "all in the name of beauty." In 1886 Harriet Hubbard Ayers launched, Recamier Toilet Preparations, Inc., the first cosmetic company in the United States. Her products claimed to "cure a bad skin and preserve a good one." Then along came six big hitters, who defined the cosmetic industry.

Helena Rubinstein was a global icon. In 1902 she started her business out with a single cream, and built a cosmetic empire making her one of the richest women in the world.

L'Oréal Paris started out in the hair color business in 1909, but the company soon branched out to include beauty products.

Mr. Max Factor founded Max Factor and Company in 1909. He specialized in makeup/greasepaint for Hollywood's most prestigious stars, and coined the phrase make-up (makeup).

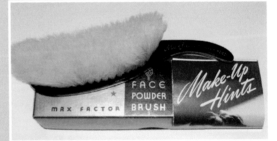

Elizabeth Arden was founded in 1910. She was a legendary cosmetic entrepreneur, and women's advocate. By 1915 Elizabeth Arden was a global brand.

Revlon was founded in 1932, and created the first glossy opaque nail enamel. By 1940 Revlon had a full line of manicure products, and began matching lips and nails.

Estée Lauder was founded in 1946 with four skincare products: Estée Lauder Creme Pack, Cleansing Oil, Super-Rich All Purpose Creme, and Skin Lotion. Today the Estée Lauder Companies include a portfolio of brands.

DO YOU KNOW YOUR FACE SHAPE?

When applying makeup, it is important to bring out your best features and minimize less attractive ones. Knowing your face shape will help you achieve your best self.

- diamond: cheeks wider than chin and forehead

- inverted triangle: heart shaped

- oval: ideally balanced

- rectangle: oblong, long and narrow

- round: round face

- square: square jawline

- triangle: pear shaped

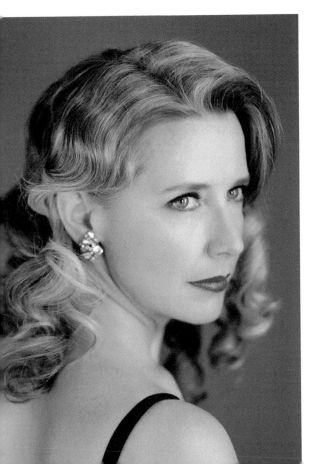

MAKEUP APPS

There are three key colors that come into play when selecting your makeup colors: eye color, hair color, and skin color. You will also want to know your undertones (the color underneath the skins surface). Skin undertones include cool, neutral and warm; neutral contains equal amounts of both cool and warm. Always start with a fresh clean face prior to any makeup application. Apply a lightweight daytime moisturizer to hydrate the skin, and use a sunscreen daily!

FACE PRIMER

A face primer will fill in your pores and create a smooth canvas for your makeup. Clinique offers six different shades in their Superprimer Face Primer. I use Colour Corrects Redness, (yellow) for my pink undertones. Face primer makes your skin look fantastic. For those who do not like to wear foundation, try using a face primer instead. You will absolutely love what this product does for your skin!

FOUNDATION

Wear foundation to even out your skin tone and protect your skin from airborne pollutants. Most foundations today include a sunscreen, which helps protect your skin, and, include other goodies as well. There are three formulations: cream, liquid, and powder. If you have dry/mature skin, you will want to use a satin finish instead of a matte. To determine your correct color, apply foundation to the jawline, if it disappears, it will blend-in perfectly with your skin tone. The secret to the right color and coverage is NOT seeing it! Most necks are a little darker than the face (thanks to sunscreen), so use a powder or bronzer to even things out a bit. When applying foundation, use a foundation brush or your fingertips. Start at the jawline and work your way up to the forehead. Blend "up and out" into the hairline. For those who want just a hint of color try using a tinted moisturizer or bronzer instead.

FACE POWDER

A powder will soften, set, and seal your makeup giving you a flawless look. Using a powder will give your makeup "staying power!" Always use a powder brush when applying face powder. Powder comes in two formulations; loose for at-home use, and cake formulation for on-the-go. Cake formulations are great for quick touch-ups and can easily be slipped into your pocket or purse! When applying loose powder, dip your brush in powder and tap gently to remove excess powder. Using a powder brush will ensure a seamless look. Using a powder-puff to apply powder may give a "mature face" a caked-on look. Helpful hint: some loose powders have microscopic sparkles, which can give your face a healthy glow and will go perfectly with the silver sparkles in your graylicious hair! So sparkle on with Lancôme Absolue Powder Radiant Smoothing Powder with micro-sparkles.

EYE SHADOW PRIMER

If you have oily eyelids or creases in your lids and can spare an extra ten seconds, you will want to use an eye primer. Using an eye primer insures that everything stays exactly where you put it! What a great invention! I recommend Clinique Touch Base for Eyes in Canvas.

EYELINER

Eyeliner emphasizes your eyes and draws attention to them. When applying eyeliner, avoid black! A black/brown or charcoal colored liner will give you a much softer, more natural look. On the top lid, any product formulation will work. If you use a pencil all you need to do is: draw a line close to the lashline, and blend with the attached sponge applicator. If you are using a cake, gel, or liquid liner; well—that's a whole different story! Making the perfect line is not always the easiest thing to do, so you will definitely want to grab a magnifying mirror for this type of application! First draw a thin line, as close to the lashline as possible, and follow-up with a slightly dampened Q-Tip to fix any mistakes. On the bottom lash, using an eye pencil will guarantee a natural look. Avoid a perfect line by using the side of your eye pencil, and blend with the attached sponge applicator. Choose between charcoal, slate, navy, violet,

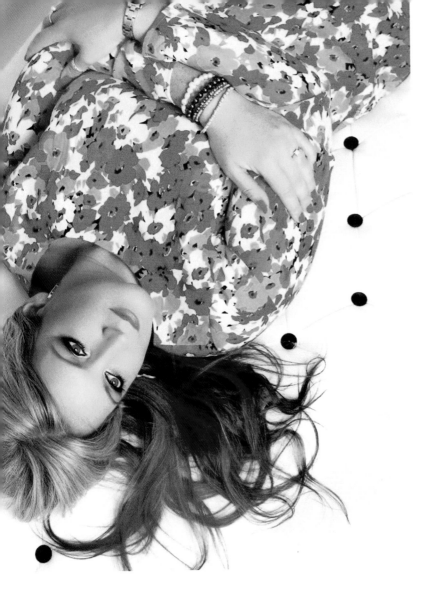

black/brown, etc. You can mix-and-match color selections and formulations, on both the top and bottom lashline. Do not make your eyes appear smaller and close them in, by drawing a continuous line across the "bottom lashes." When your lashes stop, you stop! A helpful tip: To keep your eye pencil sanitary, sharpen pencil before each use.

EYE SHADOW

If you have mature eyes, avoid powder shadows with intense sparkles. Heavy shimmers/sparkles will only emphasize lines and draw attention right to those suckers! For powder application, always apply powder shadows with an eyeshadow brush. Use soft neutral colors to insure a natural look. For eye shadow application: apply eye primer to the entire eyelid and blend with ring finger. Next, use an eye shadow brush and apply powder (highlighter/base color), to the entire eyelid; all the way up to the brow bone and blend. A highlighter will open up the eye area, and creates a "base" for the main color. Bring in the second color (main/contour color), and apply it to the crease of the eyelid and blend. Lastly, extend a tiny bit of your (main/contour color), on the "outside" corner of your eyelid; starting from the corner of the crease to the outside corner of the lashline, blend to soften. My eyes are brown, so my eye color is considered neutral, so I can wear a large selection of colors for my complementary colors! If I want my eyes to really pop, I will wear a contrasting color, like blues or blue-green. For everyday use and business attire, I recommend soft neutral colors. Helpful tip: When using a cream shadow it is imperative to use an eye primer first, otherwise the cream will accumulate in the crevasses of the lid and emphasize lines.

TIGHTLINING EYES

The tightlining procedure is used to emphasize your lashes. Do not tightline both top and bottom lashes, or it will actually make your eyes look smaller. Tightlining will make your lashes look extra thick, and will fill in any gaps between your lashes. Use a cake formulation only. Tightline the lashline only, not the waterline. If it gets on your waterline, use a clean fingertip and blink to remove. Tightlining should be done prior to mascara application. For instruction's, you can check out the many video's online. The benefit of tightlining is thicker, fuller, longer looking, lashes. Eyeliner: Laura Mercier Tightline Cake Eyeliner: Charcoal Grey.

LASH CURLER AND LASH PRIMER

Your first step to great-looking lashes starts with a lash curler. Always use a lash curler on dry, clean, mascara-free lashes. Secondly, use a lash building primer (small white fibers) to condition and lengthen your upper eyelashes, and to get the most out of your mascara. Use only a small amount of lash primer or you will end up with clumped-up lashes; do not let it dry before applying mascara. No matter what mascara you use, adding a lash primer will give your lashes that extra boost!

MASCARA

Mascara opens up the eye area and will give your eyes definition. Mascara comes in two formulations; water resistant and waterproof. Water resistant mascara is what most people wear, and can easily be removed. Waterproof mascara is used when water or tears are involved, such as weddings, break-ups, funerals, swimming, etc., and cannot be removed without a special eye makeup remover. Once you curl and prime your lashes you are ready to apply your mascara. You cannot go wrong with black mascara! To lift the eye area: emphasize the top lashes, and under-emphasize the bottom lashes. Two gray8 recommendations include: Lancôme Grandiôse: Noir Mirifique, and Maybelline the Falsies: Very Black.

CONCEALER

Using a concealer will minimize lines, hide imperfections, erase dark circles, and lighten and brighten the eye area. Be aware however, that not all concealers are created equal and formulations do vary. For hiding imperfections, apply concealer "before" makeup application. For the delicate eye area, you will want to use a very lightweight formulation. If the formulation is too heavy, the concealer will only emphasize lines instead of hide them, (that holds true for foundation also). When using concealer, you only need to use a very small amount; less is more. For the eye area, apply concealer with your ring finger in order not to stretch the delicate skin around the eye. Re-apply concealer once again (under the eye area), as a last step once your eye makeup is set. Helpful tip: If I'm going to be spending a lot of time outdoors, I use a "heavy" concealer on my brown spots for "added" protection against the sun.

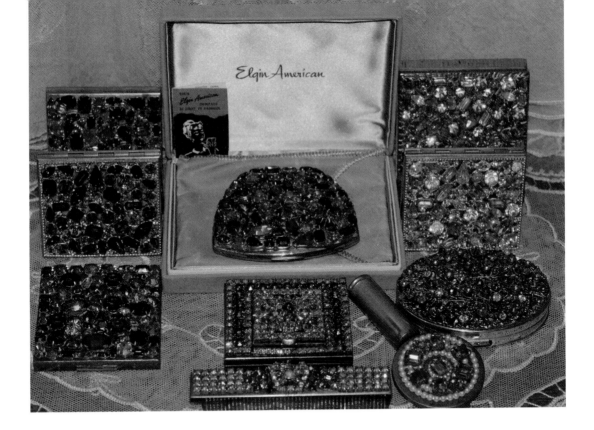

EYEBROWS

Applying color to your eyebrows should be part of your daily makeup routine, never leave home without your eyebrows on! For more information, (brows) browse through GGG's eyebrows 101.

BLUSH AND BRONZER

A little color on the cheeks goes a long way in giving your face a healthy glow. You can choose from two formulations; cream or powder, depending on your preference. To apply cream blush, blend "up and out" towards the hairline; you can build color by layering. If you have oily skin and large pores, do not use a cream formulation. For powder application use a blush brush; remember to gently tap your brush to remove excess powder before each use. Apply powder blush to the cheek area in an upward circular motion; blend into hairline with fingertips. If you have a mature skin, do not smile while applying any type of blusher, because, once you stop smiling, your blush will drop lower than it needs to be. Blush should always look natural; you don't want an obvious "pink circle" on your face! Seal cream or powder blush with a loose invisible/translucent powder. Remember if your cheek color is a "cool color" your lip color should also be a "cool color." Pinks and rose tones work gray8 with gray hair.

A bronzer can give your skin a sun-kissed glow, but choose your color wisely; too many orange faces out there! Choose a shade or two closest to your own natural skin color, and blend to insure a seamless look.

LIPSTICK

Using a lip pencil to line the lips will make them appear fuller, keep lipstick in place, and, give them definition. When picking out a lip pencil, chose a neutral color that is closest to your lipstick shade. To begin, pat on a very small amount of concealer to cover your lips; this will help the color stay true. Next, outline and fill-in the lips with your lip pencil; this will form a base and give your lipstick staying power. Apply lipstick with a lip brush; afterwards touch-ups can be easily done using the lipstick tube. Gray8 lipstick colors for cool skin tones include: raspberry, roses, pinks, and blue-reds. Remember reds can be cool, warm, and neutral. If the red is blue-based, it's cool, if it's yellow-orange based, it's warm, if it has equal amounts of warm and cool, it's neutral. Too-dark lipstick SHOUTS from the rooftop, ages you, and makes small lips appear even smaller. If ever in doubt, use a pretty pink to perk things back up!

3-MINUTE DASH-OF-COLOR MAKEOVER

Here is a 3-minute "tried and true" makeover designed for fair skin. Start your timer!

foundation: (pick one): Clinique Age Defense BB Cream Broad Spectrum SPF 30, shade (01), or Lancôme BB Bienfait Teinte Beauty Balm SPF 30, shade Porcelaine (1).

blush: (pick one): Clinique Soft-Pressed Powder Blusher: New Clover, Lancôme Blush Subtil: APlum.

eyeshadow: Neutral Colors.

eyeliner pencils: (pick one): Clinique Quickliner For Eyes: Black/Brown (11), True Khaki (05), Slate (04), and Violet (06).

lash primer: Clinique Lash Building Primer.

mascara: (pick one): Lancôme Definicils: Black, Clinique High Impact Extreme Volume Mascara: Black, Maybelline Great Lash Washable Mascara: Black, or Maybelline the Falsies: Very Black.

concealer: Lancôme Effacernes Waterproof Protective Undereye Concealer: Ivoire.

brows: (pick one): Lancôme Modele Sourcils Brow Groomer: Taupe, Lancôme Le Crayon Poudre Brow Expert: Taupe, Clinique Brow Shaper: Charcoaled (05), or Chanel Crayon Sourcils Sculpting Eyebrow Pencil: (10) Blonde Clair and (40) Brun Cendre.

lippie: (pick one): Clinique Different Lipstick: Raspberry Glace (33) or Sweet Honey (61), Clinique Chubby Stick Moisturizing Lip Colour Balm: Woppin' Watermelon (6), Clinique Butter Lipstick: Pink-A-Boo (437), or Burt's Bees Tinted Lip Balm: Hibiscus.

done! You look graylicious!

note: All the products mentioned in the 3-minute makeover are tried and true; meaning I have actually tried each one of these products!

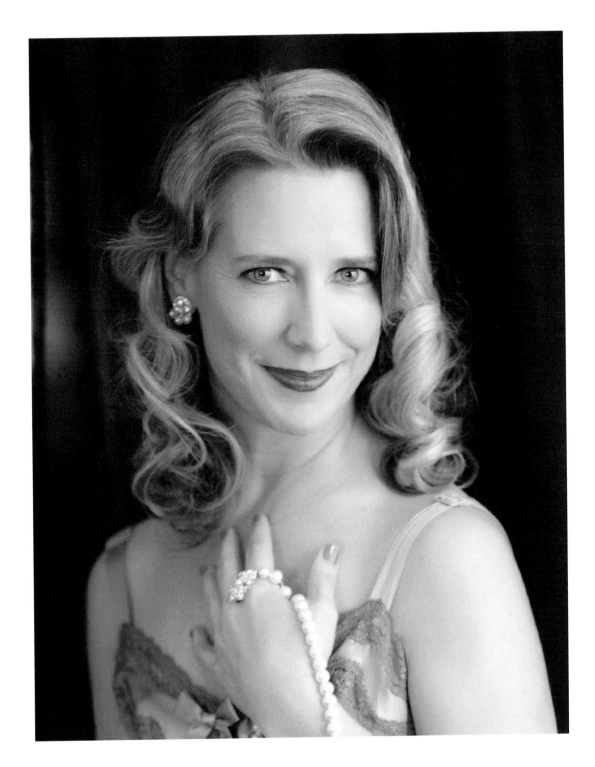

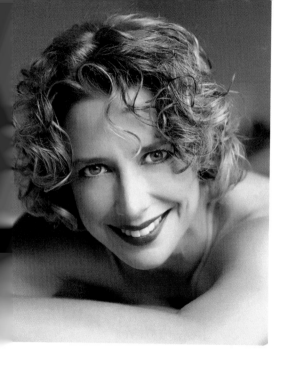

gray8 lippies

The great thing about lipsticks today, is that there is a formulation to fit everyone's needs. You can choose from 12-Hour, All-Day, Buttery, Creamy, Fade-Resistant, Feather-Resistant, Glossy, Long-Lasting, Matte, Moisturizing, Satin, Sheer, Shine, Stain, Water-Resistant, and the list goes on and on! The hard part is picking out the right shade! When choosing a lipstick, have a Beauty Advisor/Consultant apply a small amount on you; sometimes a color may appear dark, but goes on very sheer. Look in the mirror; if you suddenly go into shock—well, that means it's probably a tad too dark! LOL! Find a teasing, pleasing, shade you feel more comfortable with. A true test for choosing the correct lip color is: when you look in the mirror, where are your eyes drawn to first? If you answered lips, balance things out by adding a little more color to your face, or a little less color to your lips. You want people to look at your "entire face," not just your lips!

GGG'S FAVORITE PICKS

Burt's Bees Tinted Lip Balm: Hibiscus.
Chanel Rouge Allure: Seduisante (91).
Clinique Buttery Shine Lipstick: Pink-A-Boo (437).
Clinique Chubby Stick: Whoppin' Watermelon (06) and Super Strawberry (07).
Clinique Different Lipstick: Raspberry Glace (33) and Sweet Honey (61).
Dior Rouge Dior: Rose Taupe Tulip Pink (448).
Estee Lauder Pure Color Lipstick: Crystal Pink (03).
Lancôme Rouge In Love: Jolis Matins (106M) and Midnight Rose (377N).

MORE GRAY8 LIPPIES

Marni: "L'Oreal Color Riche: Spiced Cider (755). Revlon Super Lustrous: Smoky Rose (245)."
Meg: "Origins: Petunia (24)."
Annette: "Maybelline Baby Lips: Pink Punch (25), and Cherry Me (15)."
Chris: "Clinique Butter Shine Lipstick: Fresh Watermelon (414)."
Maxine: "Cover Girl Smoochies Lip Balm: Tweet Me (225) and Only U (270)."
Regina: "Burt's Bees Tinted Lip Balm: Hibiscus, Rose, and Sweet Violet."

Melissa: "Dior Addict (626). Lancôme Rouge in Love: Rose Sulfureuse (379N)."

Eloisa: "Revlon: Raisin Rage (630)."

Sharon: "Revlon Color Burst Lip Butter: Pink Truffle (001)."

Jodi: "Cover Girl TruShine Lipcolor: Raspberry *Shine* (455)."

Kathy: "Maybelline 24 Hour Superstay: On and On Orchid (070), Everlasting Wine (005), and Endless Ruby (030)."

Shelly: "Clinique Long Last Lipstick: All Heart (15)."

Cynthia: "Maybelline 24 Hour Superstay: Unlimited Raisin (050), and Forever Chestnut (115)."

Linda: "L'Oreal Infallible Le Rouge: Refined Ruby (337). L'Oreal Color Riche: True Red (315)."

Jo-Anne: "Revlon Just Bitten Kissable Balm Stain: Honey (001). Revlon Lip Butter: Raspberry Pie (010)."

Carmen: "Ecco Bella Flowercolor Lipstick: Claret Rose and Sangria."

Denise: "Rimmel: Amethyst Shimmer (084)."

Sheree: "MAC: Cosmo (A16). Clinique Long Last Lipstick: Berry Freeze (10)."

Deb: "Maybelline: Tinted Taupe (355). No7: Smooth Shiraz, (wear together)."

Val: "Clinique Long Last Lipstick: AL Silvery Moon."

Shirley: "Chanel Rouge Coco: Olga (422)."

Amanda: "Palladio Tinted Lip Balm: Brownie. Revlon ColorBurst Lip Butter: Lollipop (075)."

Marjori: "Lancôme L'Absolu Rouge: Boudreaux (174). Maybelline: Very Cherry (635)."

Sue: "NYX: Chic Red (516A)."

Lisa: "Clinique Different Lipstick: A Different Grape (04). Clinique Almost Lipstick: Black Honey (06)."

Mary: "Bobby Brown: Heart (13)."

Ann: "Mary Kay: Tangerine Pop, Pink Satin, and Apricot Glaze."

Cindy: "NARS: Dragon Girl (2457)."

Danielle: "Shiseido: Perfect Rouge (RS 612)."

Terri: "L'Oreal Colour Riche: Royal Red (303)."

Barbara: "Chanel Rouge Allure: Etonnante (131)."

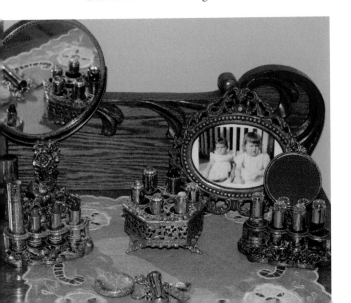

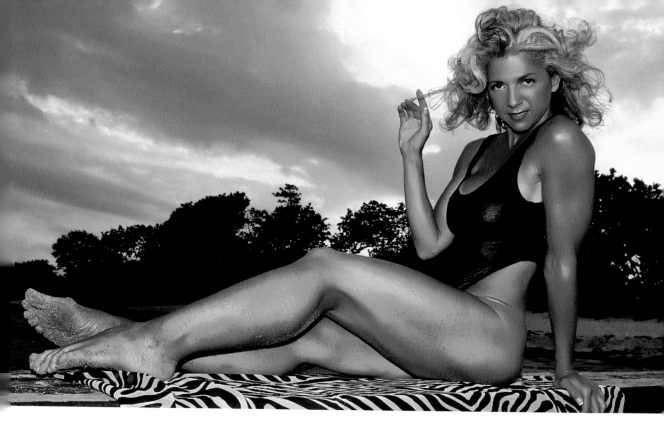

the in's & ouch of aging

GUESS MY AGE!

After high school, aging seems to take on a life of its own; prior to that, guessing someone's age was pretty easy to do. But, like they say, life happens, and genetics and lifestyle start to take over. From here on out, everyone will start to age differently. And, since everyone has their "own" perception of what a certain age should look like, well anything goes, and the guessing games begin! We love when they guess we are younger, and get mad when they guess we are older! Sometimes, we even get mad when they guess our actual age! Really? Well—don't get too mad; it's only a guess! You can ask ten different people and no doubt, get ten different answers, so just pick the answer you like best! Many times, people will guess younger because they know that is what you want to hear; otherwise, why would you be asking? I make it a habit not to play the "age game," but felt compelled to give it a try just to prove my point. I found an online site where you can guess someone's age. Let's just put it this way; you do NOT want me guessing your age! LOL! Bottom line; don't get too hung up on a guess! Age is only a number, what matters in life, is how YOU feel about YOU!

There are many variables that contribute to how a person will age.

- Genetics

- Health: (physically and emotionally)

- Lifestyle: (alcohol, smoking, drugs)

- Environment: (pollutants, sun damage, etc.)

HOW DO YOU FEEL ABOUT AGING?

Jan: "I am 62. I can honestly say that I really don't mind wrinkles, (but that could be because I don't have a lot of them yet). On the other hand, I am not a huge fan of anything sagging or drooping like my eyelids, neck, jowls, and body in general. So what does that leave? My feet? Do feet sag? LOL! I have learned that looking good doesn't have to mean 'looking younger,' it's looking good for your age! A great example of that was my mother; she always took great pride in herself, and was a beautiful woman. If I can look like my mom, and be as active and healthy as my dad is at 87, then I will consider myself pretty lucky."

Monica: "I'm 50, but will forever be 25 in my head."

Joan: "I am 66. I always thought that when you received old age pension, you were automatically old! Now it is just another number to me. Oh, there are days I feel old when my body is really sore, or I look in the mirror and see my entire body drooping, but I really don't think too much about being old; it is what it is. I find the worst part is my mind, especially when I forget something. But do I wish I was 46? Absolutely!"

Patti: "I'm 58 years young, and have never felt or looked better in my life! The systems I keep in place make it easy to move forward with grace!"

DH: "I am 57, and embrace aging naturally! No hormone replacement therapy and no medications! I have been post-menopausal for four years. I still feel sixteen, except for a rare stiff back in the morning. I think that obsessing about aging and wrinkles, actually makes for more wrinkles."

Marianne: "I am 57. For the past three years I have come to enjoy the positive aspects of aging. I love that I no longer worry anymore if my thighs are shaking or my belly is protruding. I am now comfortable in my own skin. It's not that I have given up on looking my best. I still walk and do yoga often; it's just that now when I buy an outfit, I buy it because I like it and feel comfortable in it. I've stopped worrying if I might look too fat. Now that I am retired, I have the time to learn new things, and that's been fun. Internally, I really don't think of myself as any particular age, (until I'm asked), and then I think not bad for 57! I'm really looking forward to the second-half of my life!"

Debra: "I'm 56, and started menopause at 38, with kids that were six, nine, and eleven; it was horrible! I did hormone replacement therapy for roughly three years, to ride out the worst. Wrinkles aren't such a big deal to me, but, if I ever get blood hound eyelids or a turkey neck, those may be things I may want to change. Weight can be a sore subject in particular! Beauty standards are just so impossibly 'thin.' I let my hair go natural, as part and parcel of accepting where I am in my journey through life. This is because I sincerely do not want to waste or miss, what is good about this chapter in my life. If you are chasing what the media tells you to chase; (some vision of your 25-30 year old self), you are only setting yourself up for disappointment, insecurity, and sadness. Overall, life is good in all the most important ways. I'm aware that time no longer stretches out endlessly, and that aging is inevitable; no one gets out alive!"

Marjorie: "I'm 67 and have been fighting aging with every ounce of my being. I wish I could say I have accepted it, but I haven't. This, of course, only applies to the outer aspect of aging. The inner aspect is a different story. I love it. I have learned not to take BS from anyone and that inner peace and tranquility is something I have earned and deserve."

Melissa: "I'm 59 and can't say that I worry about aging. I have been blessed with good health and good genes, so to speak. My body isn't like it was in my 30's, but I don't worry about it anymore. I try to keep fit and take pride in my appearance, but am not obsessed about it. I love my silver hair, it represents where I am in life; middle age, confident, and happy."

Benilda: "I'm 63, and have my ups and downs. I always considered myself unattractive until I hit my 40's, (that's when I started getting noticed). But when I approached 60, I began to feel invisible again. Now, I wish I would have felt better about myself when I was younger. When I was in my 40's, people thought I was in my late 20's. But now, I don't want to know what they think. The other day, I saw a photo taken by my son that showed me from the back. My heart sank because my back was broad, and my proportions had shifted. I decided to start taking better care of myself so I can feel good about myself again. I think that being a caretaker for my husband has made me question my mortality, as well."

Lori: "I am 53. I like to think of aging as 'age-less-ing.' We are bombarded with the notion that we should look as young as possible, as if aging is shameful. Quite the opposite is true; aging is a gift and an honor, not everyone gets to grow old. As we age, it does become more important to take care of ourselves. Sometimes we start to slow down and can't do as much, but we need to 'use it or lose it!' There is nothing more beautiful than a confident 50 year old lady. I choose to embrace my age, not fight it, and make the most of myself at every age. Sure, there will always be weight to lose, styles to contemplate, and criticism to withstand. But always remain true to yourself and be proud of your age!"

Kathy: "I am 58. Before I went gray, I feared aging. But now I have no fears as far as wrinkles, and bags and sags are concerned. I've always believed that it's important to take care of yourself; that hasn't changed. But I understand now, that I'm not going to get the same results as I once did. This bothered me before I went gray, but once I became more accepting of my natural hair, that acceptance spilled over into other aspects of my life. None of it bothers me now, and I'm a more content person because of it. It's not that I have developed an 'I don't care about myself attitude,' it's just that I have learned to accept that aging is all part of life. If you keep chasing what you used to be, you will never enjoy the stage of life you're in. As far as what others think, I never worried about it that much before, and I worry even less now. If I'm going where I know I will see someone that I haven't seen for a while, I tell myself to walk into the situation with joy. I don't allow my gray hair, my lined face, or my extra 25 pounds (that I need to lose), walk into the room. I allow my smile, and my joy of seeing them, to enter the room instead."

Kitty: "I'm 65, and the past five years of my life, have been better than I ever dreamed possible. It's because of who I am married to, and the support he has shown me. He encouraged me to stop coloring my hair; how smart was he? He loves my body and my face, and this in turn, has taught me to accept myself and the aging process. I am so thankful to be alive and well. I miss the energy of my youth, but I am wiser, less timid, and not afraid to be myself. I greatly appreciate my large jar of moisturizer, the older I get, the more I use LOL! I try very hard to not live in the past, but to savor each day and those I love."

Chrissy: "I am 67. Recently, I compared myself unfavorably with someone who was six years younger than me, and looking glamorous. My other half said that the difference between us was marginal, and, after all, the other woman was younger. Bless him, he meant well, but I shed a few tears. I have never felt very attractive. I was overweight when I was young, and well-meaning people used to tell me about my tendency to put on weight around my middle. By the way, this has not changed. I also always felt too tall, at five-foot-seven. Now add in the saggy jowls, arms, etc., that I have now! Okay that's most of the bad stuff! At 67, I'm not afraid to express my point of view, but I also know when keeping quiet is the best option. I feel blessed to a have such a wonderful family and six loving grandchildren!"

Annie: "I'm 62, but mentally I'm 22. I have the internal energy to continue my research and writing, but not the external energy I once had. Recently I wanted to go hiking, but unfortunately have physical difficulties now, living the lifestyle I want. But I know I need to face it, and concentrate on the things that I can do. It seems like the capacity to play and have fun wanes with the years."

Chris: "I am 63. I adore my age and mental state and find it very freeing. However, health can be challenging as we get older. It doesn't matter how old we are, only that we have good health!"

Julianne: "I am 65. I went through menopause early as well—I was under 38, and my children were ten and six. I was working full-time and had an extremely stressful job in the financial sector. I always blamed my stress problems, and insanity, on my job, but looking back, it could have been menopause. I never felt any physical issues as I did go on HRT for about ten years. As far as age, I was always told I looked young for my age. People were often shocked when they found out my age. I don't get the shocked reaction any longer, so I guess I'm looking my age. LOL! I'm very lucky that I don't have many wrinkles, but my neck is a saggy turkey looking mess. But what bothers me most about aging are the health issues; decreased energy, arthritis, vision loss, insomnia, and now hip replacements! As for energy, when I think of everything I used to accomplish as a full-time working mother, I miss the 'me' I once was. I've never worried much what other people thought, and with age, that's become even more of a benefit. I love being retired, and looking forward to this next part of my life."

Trudy: "I'm 57, but in my mind I'm 37. I don't feel 57, but I know I look it, and there are days my body reminds me. Although I carry extra weight, I've been very fortunate to have inherited my mother's genes, and at least it is evenly distributed. I enjoy exercising, and I feel it has benefited me in so many ways as I age. It keeps me flexible, makes me feel good about myself, and even has a social aspect to it. I'm learning to deal with the changes to my skin, my neck, and my face. I focus on my favorite feature, which is my eyes, and still enjoy playing with makeup. I have vowed to enjoy each year, and take care of myself, and not stress myself out too much about getting older. I'll face the challenges as I encounter them. I believe it's all about attitude. Sometimes, we are too hard on ourselves and worry too much about how others see us. But what's most important is how we see ourselves."

Mary: "I'm 68, and have never really worried about aging, but do wish my memory was better. At my age, I am sad to realize that there's not as much time left, and I still have so many things I want to see and do. I don't like my wrinkles, lines, bags, sags, and droops, but I love my silver hair and accept the rest, as part of life. I know I'll never be this young again, so why not try and make the most of it. I do wish I had more energy, and some days, I can feel that I'm getting old and realize it's so important to eat well, and exercise to keep as fit as possible. I have definitely grown in confidence as I've aged, and I don't worry about what others think so much anymore. It's so important to keep a sense of humor, and laugh as much as possible; it's an instant lift to the face and the spirit, and helps keep us young."

Kay: "I'm 64 and feel great about it. I don't like the sags and bags, but overall, my age has nothing on me! I love the freedom of not worrying about "others" opinions of me, and I only want to be true to myself. It's taken so many years to get here. I would have preferred this same freedom when I was younger."

Dawn: "I am 54. Several years ago, I might have groaned at this question, but now I can honestly say that I'm quite alright about who I am, wrinkles, gray hair, and all. I'm doing what I can to stay healthy, with a few lifestyle changes, such as, watching what I eat, exercising moderately, letting stressful things roll off my back, and laughing a lot. I'm lucky because I'm doing all this with the help of my best friend, my hubby."

Dianne: "I am 60. I don't worry about aging and feel I'm at a great place in my life right now. I graduated with a degree in Fine Arts two years ago, after following a childhood dream. I divorced my husband six years ago, after 30 years of marriage, and I'm enjoying my space and freedom. Both grown-up sons have moved to Australia and I love our visits to and from the UK. Ironically, I went gray, as I couldn't afford a hairdresser post-divorce, and now I have people comment positively on my looks almost daily; it is uplifting. I have never felt so visible, and I am forever grateful for my life."

Hillary: "I am 52. My personal view is that age is just a number and should not define you. It's not about how old you truly are, but how truly young you feel."

Viv: "I am 59. I am not too bothered about the numbers, just the aches and pains that seem to go along with them. The worst part is I need my specs to see everything, and sleep seems to be a huge challenge. My memory is appalling, and my bones ache. I started menopause at 36, with two kids under two and a six year old; it was the most awful time of my life. I truly thought I had early onset Alzheimer's. I had ten years of HRT and stopped at 46. I think menopause is one of the most horrific things, that has ever happened to me, but I came through it. What doesn't kill you makes you stronger, right? I love my job, have amazing friends, and have never been busier! I think that age brings freedom. I'm not being the slightest bit bothered about people's opinions, etc., and I just try to focus on being myself and being a good person. It's sobering, sometimes, to think that this is the end stretch, but in my head, I'm 25, so honestly, the good outweighs the bad. I'm here, and life's good."

Beth: "I'm 52, and officially menopausal. It's been a tough couple of years. I've lost all my old people, and I really wore myself out being my mother's caregiver. I think the stress of caring for her daily, all day, for almost three years, along with menopause, took its toll on my face, body, and looks. I've really been trying to take better care of myself lately. I will admit I neglected myself terribly while my mom was on Hospice. I used to be very pretty, now, not so much. Sometimes, with the weight gain and silver hair, I don't recognize myself anymore. I am considering a face lift, and some pretty dental work, I've always wanted straight teeth. I will be starting a new job in a couple of weeks. I am looking forward to that. I've been home for 22 years. Now that my kids are almost grown and mom is gone, I'm finding myself looking for another purpose. There has to be more than keeping the house clean. I don't mean to sound whiney, but I'm being brutally honest. I love my husband and sons, have a good life, and I try to focus on the positive. My health is good, but I'm more out of shape than I have ever been! I feel a little off-kilter and need to start another chapter, now I just need to figure out what that's going to look like."

Michelle: "I am 51. Just a few years ago, I swore I would color my hair until the day I died. Then I made some healthy lifestyle changes and let my hair go natural. Everyone always thought I looked young for my age, so I never really thought about aging until I stopped coloring my hair. Yes, I have the changes in my body that go along with aging, but I'm okay with it. Being and looking healthy are more important to me now, then trying to look younger than I actually am. I love who I am right now, and I don't worry anymore about what others think."

Natalie: "I am 55. Does anyone love to get old? No, I'm pretty certain no one loves aging. However, there are some of us that can see the benefits of aging. At 55, and having just finished treatment for breast cancer, I have a fresh perspective on life. There are many things I actually do love about aging, believe it or not. I love being a grandparent; it is truly the best thing for your heart. I love that I now live each day understanding what true love is, what terrible loss actually means, what true faith is, and what's really important in life. Without aging, I simply would not know these things. I believe that all we have to leave our loved ones is memories, and I plan to leave them lots of fun memories!"

Maureen: "I'm 56, and I feel aging is a blessing. I am much more confident, wiser, calmer, and less inclined to give a hoot what others think."

Catherine: "I am 42. To me, aging is inevitable. You can either fight it, or work with it. My plan is to work with it the best I can and age gracefully! I also am doing what I can to stay healthy, by staying active, drinking lots of water, and eating nutritional foods!" I have a few wrinkles around my eyes. My skin is oily, which helps keep the wrinkles away. I'll never resort to cosmetic surgery or laser treatment for wrinkles. But I do have brown spots on my face that show more in the summer. I would consider a treatment for those."

Kim: "I'm 55, and haven't felt this free in 30 years, (the age of my oldest daughter). My wonderful husband and I have raised three beautiful daughters. Our youngest is nineteen and in her second year of college. I am also a grandmother to a beautiful baby girl. I worked as an RN for years in the ICU, and know how fragile life is. I appreciate good health; I work out, eat well, and know the importance of taking good care of myself, amongst other things. A very wise friend once said, "Would you rather look great for 50, or would you rather people think you look old for 40?" I just want to be the most authentic and best version of myself that I can be. I'm proud of my age and happy to age gracefully! I've earned every wrinkle and every gray hair! No matter how hard we fight, we are all going to age. We might as well enjoy the ride!"

Barbara: "I am 62. Of course, I'm not thrilled about the wrinkles, arthritis, menopause, hot flashes, dry skin, aches and pains, lines, wrinkles, a fat ass, sagging boobs, flabby arms, jiggly thighs, chronic spine pain, loss of short term memory, and so on. Then there are the appointments with my many doctors—psychiatrist, physical therapist, bariatrician, surgeon, and endocrinologist and so on. Having had cancer, I'd rather experience all of these things than not. Salt and pepper hair, however, is one of the outward signs of aging that I'm digging. With age comes freedom to do what I want, when I want, and with whom I want. I am still with the same guy who I married in 1976. Financially, we are more than comfortable. We live in a beautiful home without a mortgage, with things of great beauty that we've collected over decades of extensive traveling. We live in a beautiful area with fabulous cars, two dogs, and five cats. We went from borrowing ten dollars from a co-worker on Fridays so that we'd have enough money for the weekend, to paying off a student loan, and paying off a business loan, to where we are today. We now can have our cake (well, figuratively) and eat it, too! Now, that's the freedom that comes with age!"

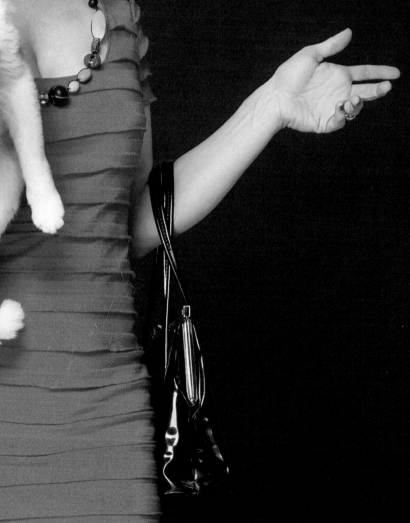

gray8
style

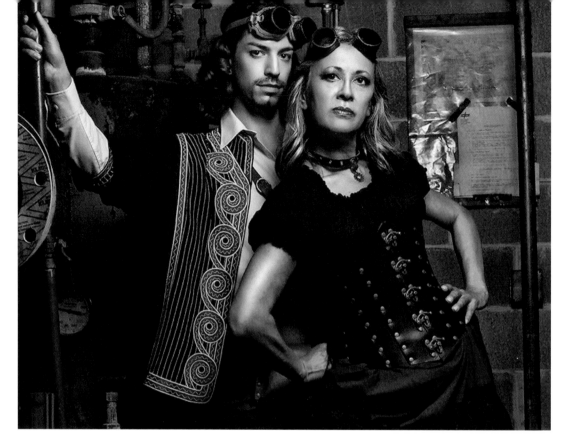

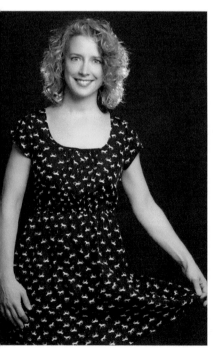

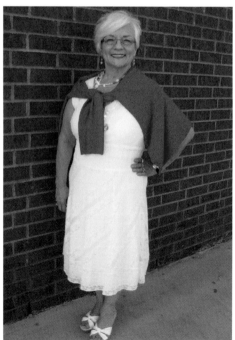

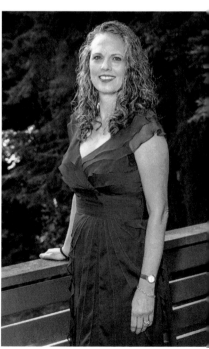

colors in my closet

Understanding the concept of color will help you create your own individual palette and complement your overall features. Familiarize yourself with the color wheel. Getting to know how color works will help you better understand color theory, and determine your best colors. The world of color can be an exciting one, and the color selections are endless! For those needing assistance with their wardrobe colors, I highly recommend "Color Your Style" and "How to Win at Shopping" by Emmy-Award Winning stylist, Davis Zyla.

There are three basic color theory categories: Primary Colors, Secondary Colors, and Tertiary Colors. The color wheel is based on three Primary Colors: blue, yellow, and red. When you mix equal parts of two Primary Colors, you create a Secondary Color. Secondary Colors are green, orange, and purple. For example: yellow mixed with blue equals green, yellow mixed with red equals orange, and red mixed with blue equals purple. Tertiary Colors are formed by mixing a Primary Color and a Secondary Color. For example: yellow (Primary) and orange (Secondary) equals Tertiary Colors.

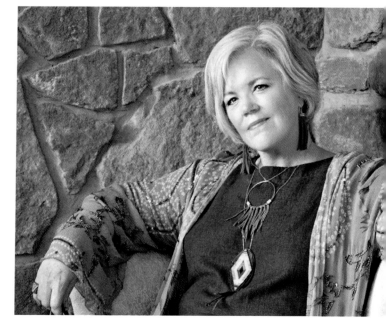

Complementary Colors are any two colors that are directly opposite each other on the color wheel. For example: red is opposite of green, yellow is opposite of purple, and blue is opposite of orange. Placed next to each other, they create a maximum contrast. Warm Colors have a yellow undertone and include variations of reds, yellows, gold, oranges, and yellow-greens. Cool Colors reflect coolness and include variations of purples, blues, blue-greens, and blue-reds. Black, silver, white, and gray are neutrals; white can be both cool and neutral, depending on the undertones.

Sometimes it's easier to gravitate towards the same old two or three go-to colors. You already know they work with your skin tone, hair, and eye color and are a safe choice. They have become staples in your closet, and you have become to rely on them. Picking out a color that already works, makes shopping a breeze! BUT what if, there were other colors that you could rely on as well? Would you be willing to give them a try? Find out what makes your skin glow, your eyes sparkle, and your hair shine bright! Wearing your best colors will not only make you look gray8, but feel gray8 too! Let's take a sneak peek inside some of your neighbors' closets and see what colors we can find!

Jan: "My favorite colors in my closet are black, charcoal gray, dark chocolate brown, dark navy, midnight blue, royal blue, cornflower blue, blue-red, royal purple, eggplant, dark forest green, dark olive green, blue-green, red-orange, dark raspberry, clear neutral pastels, certain creams, and soft white."

Trudy: "Dark purple, black, navy, red, pink floral patterns, and jewel-tones."

Melissa: "Rich clear colors like reds, purples, deep blues, white, black, and teal."

Heather: "I wear deep bold colors; black, navy, red, dark purple, etc., and accessorize with colorful scarves."

Deb: "I wear a rainbow of colors; black, white, pinks, reds, cobalt blue, yellow, and orange."

Debra: "Warm reds, olive green, golden orange, navy, denim, black, chocolate brown, caramel, and purple."

Kathy: "Purple, black, dark blue, navy blue, red, gray, and dark brown."

Kama: "My favorite colors are turquoise, raspberry, black, and gray."

Sheila: "Jewel-tones and bright colors, especially purples, teal, red, and pink, also black, white, gray, and silver."

Dianne: "Black, blue, brown, white, purple, teal and jewel-tones. I also wear black and white patterned tops."

Jessica: "My favorite colors in my closet are purple, blue, black, dark brown, and gray."

Becky: "My favorite color combo is red, white, and blue. My other favorites include: cobalt blue, navy, aqua blue, red, fuchsia, black, and silver."

Chrissy: "Black, navy, coral, dark brown, teal, turquoise, denim-blue, and touches of white and cream."

Marjorie: "My favorite colors are blues, red-orange, soft yellow, green, black, beige, and red."

Tricia: "Black, white, silver, gray, navy, denim, red, fuchsia, teal, and turquoise."

Anne: "Pink, periwinkle, turquoise, black, gray, red, coral, raspberry, and all shades of blue."

Judy: "My go-to colors are purple, magenta, red, fuchsia, black, navy, rose, pink, and lime green."

Shawn: "My favorite colors in my closet are black, pink, red, teal, and coral."

Sherry: "My favorite colors are red, black, navy, turquoise, fuchsia, and bright blue."

Kay: "Wedgewood-blue, plum, eggplant, forest green, dusty rose, gray, mauve, charcoal, brick red, teal, sage green, coral, silver, true red, olive green, deep purple, and midnight blue."

Lilly: "The colors in my closet are black, gray, red, brown, white, and lots of blue shades."

Janice: "My favorite go-to colors are black, gray, purple, hot pink, floral, red, and cool brown."

Nancy: "My favorite colors in my closet are navy, lavender, coral pink, hot pink, and white."

Jeannine: "Black, gray, purple, royal blue, navy, fuchsia, white, and dark denim."

Arlee: "Teal, black, coral, navy, peach, fuchsia. I stay away from tan, pale yellow, and green. If I happen to love a certain top in those hues, I embellish it with a scarf or a piece of chunky jewelry."

Mary: "Red, purple, fuchsia, navy, pink, and gray. I have never worn black, as it is a color I just don't like."

Joanna: "Red, black, purple, royal blue, navy blue, hot pink, gray, and white."

Donna: "My favorite colors in my closet are turquoise, black, fuchsia, navy blue, and royal blue."

Wilma: "I like white shirts with tan and denim, chartreuse, red, chocolate brown, gray, yellow, turquoise, and, of course, black is my go-to color."

Denise: "Black, gray, navy, aubergine, blue, purple, red, pink, and white."

Nancy: "My favorite colors are black, silver, magenta, cranberry, purple, and red."

Dulcy: "I like deep bold colors, like navy, black, dark brown, charcoal gray, and several shades of blue."

Bea: "Black, white, gray, red, burgundy, pink, fuchsia, purple, blue-greens, turquoise, periwinkle, bright blues, and denim."

Priscilla: "Black, silver, gray, stripes, mauve, pink, navy, and blue red."

Terri: "My favorite colors in my closet are black, red, blue, yellow, pink, and white."

Jodi: "My favorite colors are bright white, turquoise, navy, red, black, and silver."

Heike: "Black for drama and mystery; yellow for sunshine on my mind; red for power and strength; white for lightness of being; orange for fun and energy; green for accents; blue for solidity; gray for thoughtfulness; purple for an age-pride statement; and turquoise for special moments."

QUOTE FROM DAVIS ZYLA

Emmy-Award Winning stylist, and the author of *Color Your Style* and *How to Win at Shopping*.

"Nothing beats the harmony of our unique individual coloring and the combination of colors found in our eyes, hair, and skin. This palette evolves over time, and there comes a day when the shades of espresso, auburn, sand, honey, and sable found in the hair slide to gorgeous tones of silver, pewter, dove, powder and platinum. Embracing and flaunting it is true authenticity."

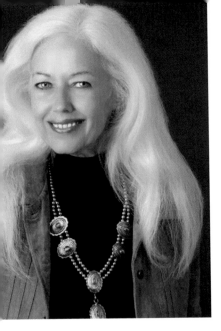

jewelry—silver or gold?

I think I decided back in high school what my best colors were. When I picked out my class ring, I chose silver over yellow gold, with a black onyx stone. Over 40 years later, silver still remains my favorite color for jewelry, along with white gold and platinum. I like my silver pieces, not only because of the way they look on me, but also because they carry with them many great memories. Jewelry is something a person collects throughout the years, and having gray hair doesn't mean you suddenly won't be wearing your gold wedding ring anymore, or your 100-year-old grandmother's ring, or anything else gold you may have tucked away.

Silver jewelry is light/cool, and gold jewelry is medium/warm. As an Esthetician, I was trained to look at hair, skin, and eye color to determine makeup colors. I use the same method for other aspects of coloring as well. Skin color and undertones together, determine the warmth or coolness of a color. Stand in front of the mirror and decide for yourself; which color is best suited for you. Remember there are no hard and fast rules when it comes to silver verses gold jewelry, and you can always mix and match! Jewelry is all about your choice and your individual style!

Basics:
- Hair color: light/medium/dark

- Eye color: light/medium/dark

- Skin color: light/medium/dark (surface color of the skin)

- Skin tone/Undertone: cool/neutral/warm (the color that shows through the skin)

Example:
- Hair color: light (white/neutral)

- Eye color: dark (brown/neutral)

- Skin color: light

- Skin tone/Undertones: (cool/pink)

- Conclusion: cool

Yes, silver looks gray8 on a cool skin tone! But "surface skin color" can change due to skin conditions and sun exposure (suntan). Yes, you will still remain a cool, because of your undertones; that remains consistent. However, now with the added color, light touches of gold will glisten on your skin as well. So now; both gold and silver jewelry look gray8 on you! That's why you can't go wrong with silver or gold jewelry! It's a win - win!

what color jewelry should a gray-haired person wear?

BY IMAGE CONSULTANT KATE LESER
http://www.themakeoverexpert.com

Do you want to accentuate your beautiful gray head of hair?

Are you looking to positively enhance your new image with just a few changes?

Imagine creating a visual presence with less of an emphasis on what you're wearing, but which has a greater impact on those around you.

Your brown/black hair once served as a frame around your face, naturally highlighting a favorite facial feature like eyes, cheeks, lips, or skin. Now that your hair is gray, silver, white, or salt and pepper, you may feel a bit washed-out. Well, that's because you've lost that frame! So, create a new frame!

Think accessories. Adding accessories is the easiest way to draw focus and interest up to your face, similar to what a frame does to a picture. The added benefit to using fun, interesting, and colorful accessories is that these pieces give new life to your existing outfits. Since high-fashion jewelry more often costs less than buying a new outfit, why not try to show off your new look with colorful and interesting embellishments?

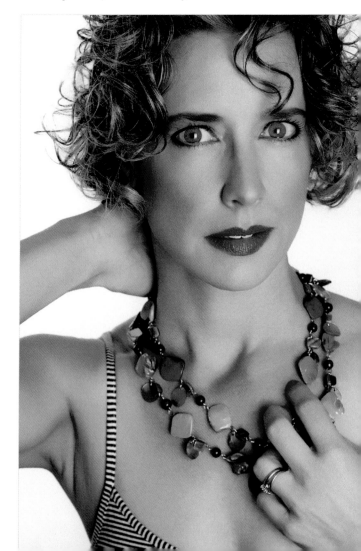

You have three key personal elements that instantly help to create your own unique style as well as a visual presence:

VALUE | FACE SHAPE | PERSONALITY

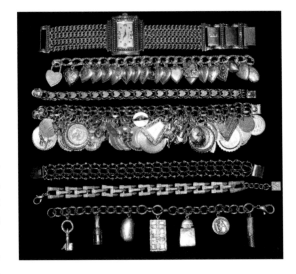

The light to dark ratios between your hair, skin, and eyes are especially important now that you are going/have gone gray. One of the easiest ways to learn about your "values" is to look at a current photo of yourself in black and white. Notice if whether you have light eyes or medium eyes. What about your skin? Is it really light or medium in relation to your eyes and hair? For example: dark eyes, light hair with light skin. Another example, light hair, light eyes with medium skin. You could also have light hair, dark eyes with dark skin.

The key is to match the value (light, medium, bright, or dark colors) of your jewelry to your own values. Matching your natural values to jewelry colors is a great way to enhance your overall look, thus drawing more attention to your face, which is what you want.

LIGHT

Your skin, hair, and eye coloring is light overall. Your best color combinations balance light to mid-range colors. Your best single colors are light to medium.

TRUE

Your skin, hair, and eye coloring is medium. Your best color combinations are medium worn with dark. Your best single colors are also medium.

VIVID

Your skin, hair, and eye coloring is mid-value to dark. Your best color combinations are bright and dark worn together. Your best single colors are bright.

CONTRASTING

Your skin, hair, and eye coloring combine lights and darks. Your best color combinations are light and dark colors worn together, with a bright accent. Your best single colors are dark and bright.

3 tips 2 looking gray8 with gray hair

BY IMAGE CONSULTANT KATE LESER

http://www.themakeoverexpert.com

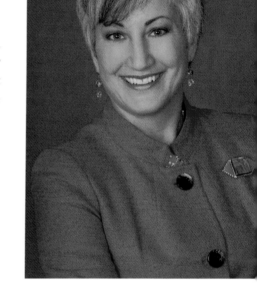

Do you think you look old?
Are you confused by what colors to wear now?
Are you willing to gain positive attention?

Your image is one of your greatest tools for success, both personally and professionally. Creating a unique image for yourself will trump any negative feelings you may have about your gray hair. Come on! Gray is the new blonde so have some fun with it!

Other than a fabulous haircut, (your built-in fashion accessory that highlights your beautiful silver locks), there are three key personal elements to wearing your gray hair proudly.

You should know your:

- Best colors

- Eye intensifier color

- Face shape

Why? Because when you wear your very best colors, necklines and accessories, people will be noticing you as a whole individual. It won't be just about your hair.

If you have never had a color analysis, or perhaps it's been a long time since you've had one. I would recommend an analysis from a respected color expert. Knowing forty of your very best colors is empowering, to say the least. Looking pretty and confident with gray hair then becomes an everyday, effortless occurrence. You begin to develop your own personal style. The guesswork in what to wear and which makeup to use is over. Your budget will be thankful!

When you get your colors done, your consultant should be able to tell you which color is the complement to your eye color. This "eye intensifier" color is the key to getting people to really hear you, because their focus will be on your eyes. For example, my eyes are a blue/gray color, and so my complement color is a lemon yellow. When I wear that particular yellow, my eyes are brighter and more intense in color. Face-to-face interactions are stronger when the other person is drawn to your eyes. You appear more approachable.

Working with your face shape is also another key point to creating your unique personal style. Similar to the color analysis, your fingerprint in Technicolor, working with the curves or angles of your face shape will be your secret weapon. It gives you the edge to stand out in the crowd—for all the right reasons!

WORD REFERENCE

So you think we made a spelling mistake? Nah!

United States	International
accessorize	accessorise
center	centre
centimeters	centimetres
color	colour
emphasize	emphasise
favorite	favourite
favors	favours
gray	grey
jewelry	jewellery
modeling	modelling
moisturized	moisturised
realize	realise
theater	theatre
traveling	travelling

gray8 reference guide/credits

going gray beauty guide

http://www.goinggraybeautyguide.com
GGG Going Gray Beauty Guide https://www.facebook.com/GGG.GoGrayGuide
GGG Going Gray Guide https://www.facebook.com/groups/1578474939074185

front book cover credits: Model: Amanda Ball - Makeup Artist: Lisa Maners - Photo credit: Guillermo Umbria http://www.guillermoumbria.com

back book cover credits: Model: Alex B. http://alex-therealdoesnoteffaceitself.blogspot.co.uk Photo credit: Anna Nicholas http://www.fashionablephotography.co.uk

back book cover credits (head shots): Models: Denise O'Neill Photo credit: White Hot Hair http://www.whitehothair.co.uk and Helen Smith Photo credit: Brian Muir Air Image Photography

jacket design by: Cathy Helms Avalon Graphics LLC http://www.avalongraphics.org

book design by: eBook DesignWorks http://ebookdesignworks.com

fashion & lifestyle illustrations: Artist Pepper Tharp http://www.peppertharp.com

inside front of book: Actress and Lifestyle Model: Marilyn Carlisle http://marilyncarlisle.com Photo credit: Anthony Dones http://www.darkroompictures.net

dedication: *The Westfall Sisters

a gray8 inspiration: *Gray8 Aunt Ruby

the end: *Bryn Junko

note: *Denotes family

going gray beauty guide 50 gray8 going gray stories

Alex B.
Age 55
London, England

Amanda Ball
Age 42
Tennessee

Anne Thomas Gerhardt
Age 49
Ohio

Becky Baldry Hansing
Age 67
Texas

Brandee Bolden
Age 36
Ohio

Breten Bryden
Age 52
Massachusetts

Carol Ann Cheatham
Age 51
Michigan

Cathy Graf
Age 55
Washington

Debra Toutloff
Age 56
Canada

Dede Watson Runnels
Age 48
Texas

Denise Buchoz
Age 57
Texas

Denise O'Neill
Age 52
Northern Ireland

Donna Johnson
Age 53
Indiana

Dulcy Checkland-Huard
Age 61
Canada

Helen Smith
Age 46
Scotland

Hillary Bitar
Age 52
Florida

Holly Barnett
Age 55
North Carolina

Janet Nuich
Age 58
Illinois

Jeanne Marie Viviani
Age 43
Florida

Jennifer Seminara
Age 44
Arkansas

Jenny Johnson
Age: 44
Minnesota

Jo-Anne Neilson
Age 56
North Carolina

Julie Fisk
Age 56
New York

Kama Frankling
Age 46
Sunshine Coast, Australia

Kate Leser
Age 53
North Carolina

Kate Mantz
Age 36
Wisconsin

Kay Jones Brooks
Age 64
Alabama

Kaylee Nuttall
Age 39
Chester, UK

Kitty Kuzak
Age 65
Ohio

Lauren Traverson
Age 23
Missouri

Leesa Travis
Age 51
California

Linda Love Atwater
Age 62
Arizona

Lois Khalafalla
Age 48
North Carolina

Lori Murray
Age 52
New York

Lynn C.
Age 54
Alaska

Marina Capello
Age 50
Italy

Melissa Dickson Fleury
Age 41
Arizona

Michelle Burge
Age 50
Ohio

Monica Gallacher
Age 45
Massachusetts

Monica Ludwig
Age 50
Virginia

Natalie Benton
Age 55
Kansas

Patsy Telpner
Age 62
Canada

Pip Bacon
Age 45
Oxfordshire, England

Ros Johnstone
Age 49
Essex, UK

Sandy Hicks
Age 53
Colorado

Sara Davis Eisenman
Age 38
California

Sharon Rogers
Age 50
Colchester, UK

Shelby Zehner
Age 56
Pennsylvania

Suzanne Henderson
Age 53
Michigan

Viv McRoy
Age 58
Lake District UK

chapter reference guide

gray8 beginnings

gray8 beginnings: (Black and White picture): Nicola Griffin Photo credit: Anna Scholz www.annascholz.com

gray8 beginnings: Alex B. Photo credit: Anna Nicholas http://www.fashionablephotography.co.uk

graylicous ride: Ayne Shore

introduction: *Jan Rogers

do you lose your identity when you go gray?: Denise Buchoz

a man's point of view: *Dale Rogers

your unique color combination: *Cheyenne Rogers Walker

gray8 color combo's: Becky Baldry Hansing, Beth Guy, Carrie Smith, Cathy Graf, Debra Toutloff, Denise Buchoz, Dulcy Checkland-Huard, Gloria (Gigi), Irene Smallwood-Bosma, Jade Jourdan, Jo-Anne Neilson, Kama Frankling, Karen Imeson, Kitty Kuzak, Lori Marshall Olson, Melissa Crossland, Peggy Scott Rabatin, and Sallee Smith

ditching the dye

ditching the dye: Alex B. Photo credit: Michael Culhane

the long & short of it: Shelly Rhea Coddington (pixie cut), and Linda G Wardle (long hair)

what's the best way 2 go gray?: Lisa Dee-Martin

skunk stripe: *MistyRogers, Lois Khalafalla, Debbie Smith, Lisa Dee-Martin, Eloisa Garoutte, and Noelle Smith

buzz cut - transition: Pip Bacon

cold turkey pixie cut - transition: Sharon Rogers

cold turkey length - transition: Amanda Meller

feathering – transition: Emily C Brandt

highlights/lowlights - transition: Dawn Hofstad, Lisa Dee-Martin, Monica Gallacher, Lisa Dee-Martin, Cathy Meinke, and Helen Smith

gray8 before & after pictures: Denise O'Neill (after picture) Photo credit: Gavin Byrne Red River Studios http://www.redriverstudios.net, Janet Nuich, Jennifer Seminara, Jo-Anne Neilson, Kathleen Hollerbach, Kitty Kuzak, Lisa Carpenter, Lois Khalafalla, Lori Marshall Olson, and Noelle Smith

gray8 gray hair

gray8 gray hair: Model: Alex B. **Photo credit:** Vanessa Mills www.vanessamills.co.uk

10 gray8 reasons 2 go gray: Alex B. **Photo credit:** Elina Pasok, Amanda Ball **Photo credit:** Guillermo Umbria, Denise Buchoz, Denise O'Neill **Photo credit:** Jonathan Ryder Photography http://jonathanryderphotography.com, Elizabeth McQuinn **Photo credit:** Rich Voorhees Studio, Hillary Bitar **Photo credit:** Jerry Hinkle http://www. shootfashion.com, Jeanne Marie Viviani **Photo credit:** Florida Polytechnic University, Julia Roberts, Pip Bacon, and Sara Davis Eisenman **Photo credit:** Jennifer Quest http://jenniferquest.net

10 steps 2 gray8 silver hair: Alex B. **Photo credit:** UGLY Models - www.ugly.org

10 gray8 products 4 shine: Amanda Ball **Photo credit:** Guillermo Umbria http://www.guillermoumbria.com

10 gray8 products 4 style: Kitty Kuzak

10 gray8 ways to wash long silver hair: Alex B **Photo credit:** Jeremy Howitt Photography: http://goo.gl/qLDOXb

10 gray8 mistakes: Cynthia Tipton **Photo credit:** Susan Bowlus Photography

10 do's & don'ts 4 hair loss: Denise O'Neill **Photo credit:** Catherine McIlkenny https://www.facebook.com/catherinemcilkennyphotographer

10 contributors & solutions 4 yellowing hair: Sharon Rogers **Photo credit:** Vanessa Mills Photographer www.vanessamills.co.uk

gray8 gray hair: Amanda Ball **Photo credit:** Guillermo Umbria, Denise O'Neill **Photo credit:** White Hot Hair, Helen Smith **Photo credit:** Brian Muir Air Image Photography, Hillary Bitar **Photo credit:** Jerry Hinkle http://www. shootfashion.com, Irene Smallwood-Bosma **Photo credit:** Steinman Photography/John and Betty Elder-Steinman, Jade Jourdan, Julia Roberts, Julie Fisk, Kay Jones Brooks, Kori Spence Hendrix **Photo credit:** Steve Riley Pictures http://www.steverileypictures.com, Lori Marshall Olson, and Michelle Burge

gray8 curly hair advice: by Curly Hair Specialist Scott Musgrave. Author and Founder of Curly Hair Artistry http://www.curlyhairartistry.com and MagiCurl Blog http://www.scottmusgravehair.com

what a gray8 question!: Denise O'Neill **Photo credit:** White Hot Hair - will I still look sexy with gray hair?: Amanda Ball **Photo credit:** La Photographie Nashville http://www.laphotographienashville.com

50 gray8 going gray stories

50 gray8 going gray stories: Denise Buchoz

gray8 skincare & makeup

gray8 skincare & makeup: Amanda Ball Photo credit: La Photographie Nashville http://www.laphotographienashville.com

the skinny on skincare: Alex B. Photo credit: Vanessa Mills Photographer www.vanessamills.co.uk and beauty sleep & skin: Amanda Ball Photo credit: La Photographie Nashville

eyebrows 101: eyebrow Illustration by: Debra Toutloff - eyebrow favorites: Amanda Ball Photo credit: Guillermo Umbria - over-tweezing eyebrows: Helen Smith Photo credit: Brian Muir Air Image Photography

gray8 makeup apps: Amanda Ball Photo credit: La Photographie Nashville - makeup apps: Kaylee Nuttall - 3-minute dash-of-color: Amanda Ball Photo credit: La Photographie Nashville http://www.laphotographienashville.com

gray8 lippies: Amanda Ball Photo credit: Guillermo Umbria http://www.guillermoumbria.com

the in's & ouch of aging: Model/Actress: Victoria Marie http://youtu.be/4Z8RuFWX2gs Photo credit: Rob C Photography https://www.facebook.com/robert.c.hall

gray8 style

gray8 style: Amanda Ball Photo credit: Guillermo Umbria http://www.guillermoumbria.com

looking gray8 4 a date!: Steampunk Model: Irene Smallwood-Bosma - Makeup Artist: Emmy Lindgren - Male Model: Anthony Renaissance Murray – Photo credit: Chuck Coleman http://chuckcolemaninc.com

looking gray8 4 a date!: Amanda Ball Photo credit: Guillermo Umbria, Becky Baldry Hansing, Cathy Graf, Cynthia Tipton, Dawn Morgan, Denise Buchoz, Denise O'Neill Photo credit: Gavin Byrne Red River Studios, Hillary Bitar Photo credit: Jerry Hinkle, Jeanne Marie Viviani, Julie Fisk, Kaylee Nuttall Photo credit: Chantelle Rowley http://chanteller.wix.com/photography, and Pip Bacon

colors in my closet: Cathy Hamilton quote by: Davis Zyla http://www.davidzyla.com

jewelry - silver or gold?: Elizabeth McQuinn Photo credit: Rich Voorhees Studio http://www.voorheesstudio.com

what color jewelry should a gray-haired person wear?: Article by: Image Consultant Kate Leser http://www.themakeoverexpert.com - Model: Amanda Ball Photo credit: Guillermo Umbria

3 tips 2 looking gray8 with gray hair: Article by: Image Consultant Kate Leser Photo credit: Steven Whitsitt http://www.whitsittphoto.com

gray8 reference guide

gray8 reference guide: Want more going gray stories? Check-out **going gray beauty guide 40 gray8 going gray stories:** Book cover credits: Actress and Lifestyle Model: Marilyn Carlisle http://marilyncarlisle.com - Makeup Artist: Sandy Maranesi - Photo credit: Anthony Dones http://www.darkroompictures.net

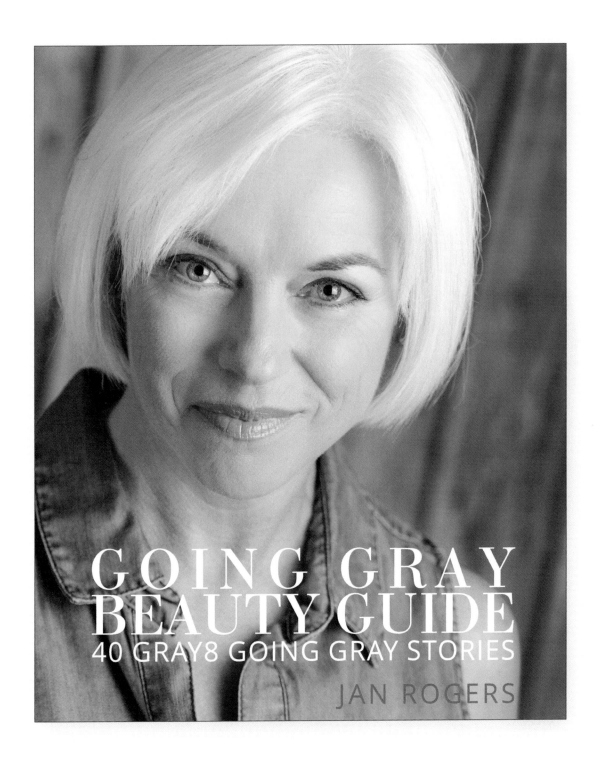

GOING GRAY
BEAUTY GUIDE
40 GRAY8 GOING GRAY STORIES

JAN ROGERS

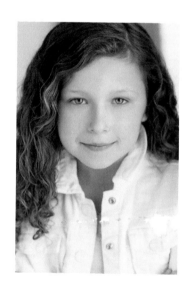

the end